Ageing and the Care of Older People in Europe

Richard Hugman

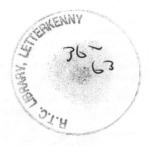

Consultant Editor: Jo Campling

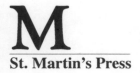
St. Martin's Press

First published in Great Britain 1994 by
THE MACMILLAN PRESS LTD
Houndmills, Basingstoke, Hampshire RG21 2XS
and London
Companies and representatives
throughout the world

A catalogue record for this book is available
from the British Library.

ISBN 0–333–58748–0 hardcover
ISBN 0–333–58749–9 paperback

Printed in China

First published in the United States of America 1994 by
Scholarly and Reference Division,
ST. MARTIN'S PRESS, INC.,
175 Fifth Avenue,
New York, N.Y. 10010

ISBN 0–312–12193–8

Library of Congress Cataloging-in-Publication Data
Hugman, Richard, 1954–
Ageing and the care of older people in Europe / Richard Hugman.
p.   cm.
Includes bibliographical references and index.
ISBN 0–312–12193–8
1. Aged—Care—Europe.   2. Ageing—Social aspects—Europe.
I. Title.
HV1480.H84   1994
362.6'3' 094—dc20
                                                            94–7205
                                                            CIP

For my parents
who are pleased to say they are
learning to grow older disgracefully

Contents

List of Tables

Preface and Acknowledgements

As we approach the end of the twentieth century one of the most noticeable features of advanced industrial society is that of an increase in the numbers of older people, as well as of the proportions of older people within the overall population. This phenomenon has generated both a growing general interest in ageing and old age and the development of gerontology, bringing together a variety of disciplines in an applied field of enquiry. There has been an accompanying increase in the number of research reports and other texts dealing with different aspects of ageing. For the student of old age there is now a wealth of material, especially that published in English. So, why another book about older people?

The main reason for writing this book is that, although much work has now been done with regard to ageing and old age, for the most part it tends to concentrate on specific national contexts. At a time when Europe increasingly (and however falteringly at times) is becoming an integrated society in which economic, political, cultural and social exchange across national boundaries is ever more important, it becomes necessary to find ways of crossing frontiers in respect of all issues. Ageing, the place of older people in our societies and the care provided for those older people who require it raise important questions for all European countries. Gerontological work from North America has tended to dominate discussions and there is still a relative lack of dialogue between European countries on this topic, although this is now being addressed in developments such as the European Community (EC) Observatory on Ageing, Eurolink Age, and work undertaken by both the Council of Europe and the Commission of the European Community.

This book concentrates on comparative perspectives within Europe and considers the implications of the social construction of and responses to old age in the various European countries. Both the diversities and the commonalities between the different parts of Europe provide a rich background against which to further develop the distinctively European contributions to understanding old age and the place of older people in society. One example of this is the theoretical approach based on political economy, grounding social gerontology in a structural analysis of the context in which old age is perceived and experienced. Indeed, as I argue in some detail, this approach provides a cogent underpinning to such debates, and, moreover, it is one which derives from the traditions of European social science. For this reason, in the early chapters I focus on more theoretical aspects, of how ageing and old age may be understood socially, before proceeding in the later chapters to examine historical and contemporary evidence about the types of response which have been made to older people in the fields of health and welfare.

In writing this study I have been encouraged by contact with a range of colleagues who share an interest in a European perspective on ageing. In particular, fellow members of the research group on the family care of older 'elderly people' funded by the European Foundation for the Improvement of Living and Working Conditions (co-ordinated by Robert Anderson) have provided much inspiration, most especially my colleagues at the Lancaster University, Janet Finch and Joy Carter, who formed the United Kingdom group on the project. This book, however, is much broader than that specific topic and seeks to develop an understanding of ageing and old age along several dimensions, placing questions of the care provided for older people within a wider context.

The completion of this text has benefited also from the critical scrutiny of Joy Carter, Jennifer Mason, Liz Mestheneos and Judith Triantafillou, each of whom have read and commented on sections of drafts, and Susan Tester who read it all. Undoubtedly it is the better for their advice, and any remaining weaknesses are entirely my own responsibility. Irini Charitou gave invaluable assistance with translation and my own struggling grasp of Greek; John Sawkins also helped with some translation. Finally, I owe thanks to Frances Arnold and Jo Campling for their encouragement and support, without which this book would not even have been started.

RICHARD HUGMAN

1

Ageing in European Society

Introduction

An ageing European population

Ageing populations are a global phenomenon. All industrialised and most industrialising countries show the same trend, which is made up of three factors:

1. A growth in the *proportion* of people aged over 65 years;
2. An increase in *absolute numbers* of older people; and
3. Improvement of *life expectancy* at birth.

Such changes are seen gradually in some countries and rapidly in others. However, the broad phenomenon of an ageing population is to be found all across Europe (Grundy and Harrop, 1992). Indeed, it may be said that it was in some European countries, most notably France, that ageing societies of the twentieth century first became evident (Stearns, 1977; de Jouvenal, 1988).

An ageing European population raises questions about the definition of old age, about the experiences of older people and their place in society, and about appropriate ways in which the needs older people who have problems of health and welfare can be met. Who do we think of as 'older people'? What does it mean to be an older person in Europe? How do European societies perceive and respond to the needs of older people?

In this book such questions about ageing in Europe will be examined in relation to the forms of social responses to old age which have developed, especially in recent decades. This discussion will focus partly on social and cultural factors which set the social boundaries of old age. Also, following the long traditions of social welfare in some European countries, we shall explore the specific issues of developing health and welfare services, and the contemporary debates about the forms which these should take.

1

In particular this book addresses the question of ageing in a European context, drawing on perspectives which make connections between the countries of the European Community (EC) in the early 1990s, the countries of Scandinavia and those of Eastern Europe. Europe is not only ageing, it is also, at the end of the twentieth century, changing dramatically. The original number of countries in the EC has doubled from six to twelve, a political grouping which appears likely to be the core of the development of European identity into the next century. Around that 'core' there is the looser grouping of the Council of Europe, the 'Europe of 25' (which includes Scandinavia, Mediterranean nations – including Cyprus and Turkey – and some states of Eastern Europe) (Council of Europe, 1991a, p. 3). In some cases former colonies and colonial powers have become partners. Moreover, the gradual integration of Europe which has followed from these changes has an impact upon the social policies and wider patterns of life in each individual country. For example, there is greater migration for employment between European countries, not only those of the EC, while increased affluence in the North has meant some migration to the South by people seeking a warmer climate in which to live. It is a new Europe in which populations are growing old.

As the phenomenon of ageing has become more apparent there has been a parallel development in studies of and writing about ageing and old age. In recent years there may be said to have been a mushrooming of literature about old age, especially in the English language. This has been influenced in part by the emergence of 'gerontology', originally in North America, as a multidisciplinary field bringing together anthropology, biology, economics, geography, history, politics, psychology and sociology as well as the professions of law, medicine, nursing, the remedial therapies and social work (Bond *et al.*, 1990). This is not say that European scholars had previously totally neglected the issue, as demonstrated by the work of Rosenmayr and Köckeis (1963), Townsend and Wedderburn (1965) or de Beauvoir (1977). Yet the extent to which ageing and the life of older people has been of concern in European writing has only approached North American proportions in recent years (see, for example, the comments of various contributors to the encyclopaedic collection edited by Palmore, 1980). The uneven development, or non-existence, of geriatric medicine as a speciality in some European countries is an illustrative example of the relatively recent growth of gerontology as a whole (Hunter, 1986).

It is my intention in this book to focus quite specifically on the evidence and analysis concerning European older people. At times it will be appropriate, or even necessary, to refer to literature concerning other parts of the world. For example, there are clear areas of similarity with other developed countries, such as Japan or the USA, and possible inferences to be drawn from a wider comparison. However, it is the intention in this book to focus specifically on the peculiarities of the European context. The increasing emergence of a *European* identity which, although not immutable, is setting the social, economic and political agenda into the next century. By locating a discrete analysis of the experiences of and responses to ageing and old age within the limits of this one continent they may be grasped more accurately. The centrality of such historical and cultural factors will be made apparent in the following analysis.

Furthermore, this book addresses areas of *social* gerontology rather than gerontology as a whole. This reflects a disciplinary division of the type identified by Victor (1987) and Bond *et al.* (1990). Victor points to three reasons why a social perspective on ageing and old age is of crucial interest at the present time:

1. Ageing as a process can be addressed from biological or psychological perspectives but the definition of old age as a life stage remains a social construction;
2. The impact of biological and psychological ideas about ageing are incorporated into general social attitudes and *in this respect* may be constituted as appropriate subjects of a social gerontology; and
3. As the pertinence of inquiries into ageing and old age is derived to a large extent from demographic change, which is a social phenomenon, then a social investigation is an appropriate way to proceed (Victor, 1987, pp. 27–8).

This is not to argue that there is a specific body of theory uncontestably regarded as 'social gerontology'. Fischer's observation that social gerontology exists as a confluence of social sciences, as an applied social science, remains appropriate (Fischer, 1978, pp. 194–5).

Fischer also assigned to social gerontology the task of challenging the prejudicial myths which may be said to have grown up around social perceptions of ageing (Fischer, 1978, p. 195). Another, more critical view is expressed by Fennell *et al.* who argue that, despite an explicit intention to confront prejudice, social gerontology may have reinforced negative attitudes through an unintended emphasis on old age as a 'problem', in the everyday rather than the theoretical sense, and reinforcing images of old people as 'pitiable' through a concentration on negative aspects in the lives of older people (Fennell *et al.*, 1988, pp. 6–12). This is an issue on which I shall touch at several points in the following discussion. In this introductory chapter I want to consider in more detail questions of who 'older people' in Europe are by examining the definition of old age and the circumstances faced by older people, within a social gerontological framework. This discussion will then be developed in subsequent chapters and the conceptual relationship of old age to social need will be explored.

Ageing and social definition

For the most part the boundary between 'middle age' and 'old age' is one which shifts between different situations. De Jouvenal summarises the prevailing view in assigning to 'old age' the normal demographic classification of people aged 65 years and over, 'whatever may be their actual situation in terms of professional activity or state of health' (1988, p. 6). In other words, such a figure is taken as a relatively arbitrary but standardised measure which may be applied to everyone.

Yet the age of 65 as the demarcation of old age is not entirely arbitrary, as we will see in more detail in Chapters 2 and 3. It is a reflection of the most widely used age criterion in industrialised societies for the receipt of retirement pensions. In this sense it cannot be completely separated from the issue of 'professional activity'. Across all the countries of Europe there is a high level of probability that a person aged over 65 years will have retired from full-time paid employment, and most people in this age group will be eligible for some type of pension *on grounds of age alone* (Johnson and Falkingham, 1992).

Another plausible perspective would be to fix a standard comparative measure, not from the more usual expectations of retirement but from the known incidence of the relationship between increasing age and increases in levels of disability and illness. If this were to be done, the figure of 75 years would appear to be most appropriate as it is within the over-75 age group that increased disability and ill-health become identifiably correlated with chronological age (see, for example, Briggs, 1990). Such an approach has actually led to the demarcation of 'older elderly people' as a term with currency in social analysis and policy responses (see, for example, Jani-Le Bris, 1992).

Both these approaches demonstrate the social nature of the definition of old age. People may not stop working at the age when they could receive retirement pension; indeed, there is much evidence that many older people do continue to work into the age of normal retirement (International Labour Organisation, 1986). Although the proportions have declined over the last thirty years, and in some instances paid employment was maintained because of low pensions or ineligibility, the figures also suggest a continuing interest on the part of some older people to continue working (see, for example, Florea, 1979; Hrynkiewicz *et al.*, 1991). In addition, there are laws or regulations in some countries or in some professions which require a person to retire irrespective of their wishes or abilities. In that sense, the average age of retirement as a definition of old age is *socially normative* rather than being neutrally descriptive. It describes what exists, but this is a reality which is the outcome of a developing view that older people *should* not work.

Similarly, if levels of disability or ill-health are taken as a measure of older old age, these too should be treated with some caution. Although this is the age group in which the incidence of needs arising from these causes rises sharply (Anderson, 1992), there is a tendency to concentrate on this aspect of life over 75 years of age. The fact that it is only a minority of people in this age group at any one time who have degrees of disability or infirmity such that they require help in daily living may be ignored (see, for example, Office of Population Censuses and Surveys, 1988). Moreover, further divisions can be made, such as that between people under and over 80 years or 90 years of age, in which other age-related factors may be identified. These include disability, life circumstances such as living alone, and gender ratios following from differentials in the mortality rates of men and women (Synak, 1987a; de Jouvenal, 1988; Parker, 1990; Power, 1990; Seale, 1990).

For these reasons, any attempt to demarcate 'old age' in strictly chronological terms is fraught with difficulty. At the same time, the age groupings to which I have referred do have a degree of common currency throughout the industrialised world. The categories 'over 65 years' and 'over 75 years' are utilised throughout gerontological study as a means of ensuring comparability (an issue to which I will return in Chapter 2). Therefore these are the definitions of older people which I will draw on in the following discussion, although at various points the limitations of such definitions and their relevance to ageing and the lives of older people in Europe will be made explicit. For these reasons also, the terms 'older people' or 'elderly people' will be used as consistently as possible to express both the relative identity of the people in question and that they are people of whom their age is but one characteristic among many. Age, however, is the primary concern of this discussion.

Ageing and social need

If the demarcation of specific chronological stages in the life-cycle is to be seen as a social construction, why then should we be concerned with the study of 'old age' and 'older people'? Would not a critical approach seek to transcend this characterisation by bridging age boundaries in other forms of enquiry into the social life of all adults, for example in gender relations, race and racism, ethnicity and culture, social class, employment and consumption patterns, health and welfare and so on?

This is, in part, the gist of the arguments of Johnson (1976) and Fennell *et al.* (1988) when they suggest that greater attention should be paid to the whole range of experience in later life, including the exotic and the mundane along with the problematic aspects of ageing. In this way the whole range of ageing and old age becomes part of the legitimate field for enquiry, and each aspect of ageing may be understood in the wider context. Indeed, the importance of problematic aspects of old age become more clearly highlighted in comparison to those features which may be regarded as positive.

Yet at the same time it should be remembered that social gerontology has developed from a concern with the problems of older people. Because of the historical construction of old age, parts of the ageing European population do face experiences of poverty, poor housing, isolation, neglect and so on. Studies have suggested repeatedly that the majority of older people experiencing these needs do so because they are over a certain age (Townsend and Wedderburn, 1965; de Beauvoir, 1977; Fogarty, 1986; Walker, 1986a, 1990). To say that old age is a social construction does not deny its power or the extent to which it is woven into contemporary European social structures and relationships as a taken-for-granted assumption about human life (Giddens, 1991).

To this extent the generally perceived 'problem' of the form, types and extent of need in old age is an appropriate 'problematic' for social science, forming the basis of questions about what is happening in European society (Mills, 1970; Goffman, 1975; Rein, 1976). The differentiation of old age as a distinct phase of the life-cycle is inherently bound up with the perception of later life as time in which problems are likely to increase and the social organisation of old age itself appears to be the origin of many of these issues (Walker, 1981, 1986b). So to investigate the social dimensions of ageing must be to enquire about the way in which social needs are perceived in age-related terms and the forms of social response which have developed around such perceptions. It is appropriate therefore to focus in part on the welfare structures and practices which have been created in different European countries. This focus will form the major emphasis of the later chapters of this book. In so doing I am aware of the risk that such an approach reinforces the equation of old age and dependency. However, to the extent that ageism, the systematic discrimination of people on the grounds of their age (Itzin, 1986), may lead to the inappropriate bracketing of all older people as 'dependent', it leads at the same time to the marginalisation of those issues concerning older people, simply because they are older. This is a contradiction which cannot be avoided.

Ageing and social divisions

Older people in European society are therefore not to be regarded as a homogeneous mass but as a diverse group of people who may have only one characteristic in common – their age. On what grounds may divisions be identified within the broader grouping of older people?

The first relevant characteristic it is necessary to recognise as it relates to later life is that of sex. The Eurostat demographic data in 1991 showed that the greater life expectancy of women compared to men is a global phenomenon. Selected figures for European countries are given in Table 1.1, which shows that women may live, on average, between 5.0 and 9.5 years longer than their male co-nationals.

The figures also show a general tendency for life expectancy at birth to be above 70 years for the average European; only men in Portugal do not appear to quite share this longevity. Yet overall the figures do not demonstrate much geographical difference in life expectancy, with a variation for women of 3.7 years and for men of 4.8. What is most apparent is that women in all countries on average are longer-lived than their male counterparts.

What the figures do not reveal is the extent to which length of life is related to quality of life. A major factor in this respect is that of poverty,

TABLE 1.1   *Life expectancy at birth, EC countries, 1990*

	Men (years)	Women (years)
Belgium	72.4	79.0
Denmark	72.0	77.7
France	72.5	80.7
Germany	72.6	79.0
Greece	72.6	77.6
Irish Republic	71.0	77.0
Italy	73.2	79.7
Luxemburg	70.6	77.9
The Netherlands	73.7	79.7
Portugal	68.4	77.9
Spain	73.2	79.8
United Kingdom	72.2	77.9

Source: Eurostat, 1991.

which several studies have shown to be prevalent among older people
(Walker, 1986a, 1987, 1990; Victor, 1987; de Jouvenal, 1988; Laczko,
1990). Not only are older people more likely to be poor people than are
their younger fellow citizens, but poverty is usually associated also with
gender and with increasing age (Synak, 1987a; Walker, 1987; Dieck, 1990;
Laczko, 1990; Siim, 1990; Széman, 1992). For this reason the issues of
retirement and pensions will be examined in more depth in Chapters 3 and
4, and linked to the question of gender. The connections between poverty
and social class will be explored in relation to conceptualisations of old age
and its emergence as a social category.

Not only are older people divided by gender, nationality and social class,
but there are also racial and ethnic distinctions which must be recognised.
De Jouvenal's demographic review in the late 1980s (1988) provides statistical evidence of immigration, showing that in 1985 there were approximately 7.3 million people in total resident in EC countries who originated
from outside the EC. In addition, there are individuals of ethnic minorities
born in EC countries who are not included in such figures, who with
immigrants may be divided from the mainstream of European society
though racism and cultural oppression (Anwar, 1979; Brittan and Maynard,
1984; Barker, 1985; Evers and Olk, 1991). Even in former colonial countries, such as France, Germany and the UK, where immigration has been
greatest, ethnic minority populations are a relatively small proportion of
the total. Older people in ethnic minority groups are an even smaller proportion. For example, in the UK, people aged 60 or over (another different
categorisation) form 7 per cent of people of Caribbean descent and 2 per
cent of people of Asian descent, compared to approximately 20 per cent of
the population as a whole (Office of Population Censuses and Surveys,
1991). However, relatively little attention has been paid by gerontologists
to this particular issue.

The lack of impact of racial and ethnic divisions can be seen in the
extent to which this minority within minorities is obscured to policy
makers and professionals (Norman, 1985; Rooney, 1987). Moreover,
ethnic minorities are more likely than their white counterparts to have
experienced other forms of discrimination, of gender and of social class
(Brittan and Maynard, 1984). For these people, therefore, old age may
represent an aspect of multiple marginalisation in a society which has,
perhaps against expectation, become a homeland (Anwar, 1979; Norman,
1985). I will return to these issues at various points in the following
chapters.

Other divisions of social structure may also be identified. Disability has
been discussed above; this is a major issue for some, but not all, older

people. Until very recently sexuality, in particular active sexuality, whether heterosexual or homosexual but especially the latter, had been a topic neglected in relation to ageing (Jerrome, 1990). Then there are religious diversities, psychological differences and biological variations which in older age reflect only the wider social distinctions which can be seen in every age group. The list of factors is extensive.

There is therefore no average European older person. Older people in Europe, as with younger people, represent a considerable diversity. At the same time, there is a common range of social factors and perceptions through which old age as a phenomenon is constructed. These have formed the basis for the emergence of general theoretical approaches to ageing and old age which seek to account for the experience of later life. In particular, three main approaches can be identified:

1. The modernisation thesis;
2. Demographic explanations; and
3. The political-economy perspective.

In the next section of this chapter I will outline these approaches and consider their utility as the basis for further discussion. The three approaches will be addressed separately as they provide contrasting explanations for the development of thinking about old age. However, some points of overlap will also be identified and I will consider also the extent to which a degree of complementarity seems necessary.

Theoretical Approaches

Modernisation

The modernisation explanation of ageing and old age in contemporary society has been articulated most clearly by Cowgill and Holmes (1972). From a cross-cultural comparison they concluded that there are eight universal factors in the construction of old age, and they identified a further twenty two aspects in which variation between different societies is observable (Cowgill and Holmes, 1972, pp. 311–3). In summary, their conclusions are that as societies industrialise, urbanise and so become more complex, the numbers of older people can be seen to increase. There is then a related decline in the status and prestige of old age arising from changes in social roles and relationships, especially individualisation. These changes have both psychological and social impact on older people, and can be seen in economic, religious, political and cultural areas of life (Cowgill, 1972). They relate also to kinship and family structures.

Theoretically, despite the apparent centrality of industrialisation as key factor in the modernisation process, this concept is based on two premises:

(a)   that all societies develop 'teleologically'; that is, in an evolutionary progression; and
(b)   that the major determinant of change is cultural (Achenbaum and Stearns, 1978; Fischer, 1978).

These two premises are expressed more explicitly in Fischer's (1978) identification of eight indicators of change in the status of older people in the USA (especially the north-east) from the eighteenth century onwards:

1. The replacement of age by ability to pay as a determinant of seating patterns in chapels and meeting houses;
2. Mandatory retirement ages for officials, including judges, introduced from 1777;
3. A tendency to overstate age in the eighteenth century, replaced by tendency to understate age by the nineteenth century;
4. A change from fashion orientated towards older people to that orientated towards youth;
5. Language of respect towards older people gradually replaced by language of denigration;
6. Changes in the representation of the heads of households, for example in paintings, literally placing them on the same plane as members of other generations as opposed to 'above';
7. The growth of 'partible' inheritance (that is, which can be divided); and
8. A decline in the practice of naming children after their grandparents.

Fischer also notes that some of these changes are gendered, for instance in claims of age (3), heads of households (6) and patterns of inheritance (7) which, at least implicitly, tended to exclude women.

However, both the assumptions behind the concept of modernisation have been questioned empirically and theoretically. With regard to the evolutionary and universal character claimed for the concept, Achenbaum and Stearns point to the extensive critique which has been developed, demonstrating its ethnocentric and a historical nature (Achenbaum and Stearns, 1978, pp. 307–8). They argue that while there is a plausible basis for using the terms 'modernisation' and 'westernisation' synonymously, there is no foundation for the equation of 'modernisation' and 'development' which is found within the literature. This appears to arise from the uncritical use of a differentiation between 'industrialised' and 'primitive' cultures and social structures which have subsequently been widely criticised in social anthropology (Asad, 1973). The anthropological data on which Cowgill and Holmes drew were, in that sense, indicative of a 'Western industrial' model of ageing and old age (compared to a variety of 'non-industrial' or 'developing' models). On this basis it becomes necessary to ask whether the differences between cultures and social structures might not be as important as the similarities, and whether all industrialised societies can be treated as a homogeneous group concerning the construction and experience of ageing (Achenbaum and Stearns, 1978, p. 308).

Taking this criticism further, Gruman (1978) has argued that the philosophical roots of modernism, which he identifies as 'positivism' (the primacy of material facts devoid of the values which give them meaning) and 'historicism' (historical change viewed as evolutionary progress), have served to create an oppressive social categorisation of later life as old age. This can be seen in the functional 'ages of man' (*sic*) models which permeated European thought and became institutionalised in the positivist natural and social sciences of the late nineteenth and early twentieth centuries (Gruman, 1978, pp. 372–4). In other words, the idea that human life could be understood in discrete stages (itself derived from classical thought) resonated with struggles to make sense of and manage the demands of a rapidly changing and increasingly complex industrial society. In this sense Gruman recognises the historically specific nature of modernism as an explanation for contemporary old age.

The other premise of the modernisation theory is that of the primacy of cultural factors. There are two respects in which this emphasis may also be seen to be misplaced, at least in its more extreme form, as evidenced by Fischer's analysis (1978). In the original version, Cowgill (1972, p. 10) points to industrialisation, and specifically the associated practice of retirement, as a major factor in the modern construction of old age. Gruman (1978) also demonstrates the way in which cultural aspects of 'old age' are moulded within a culturally specific context. This is echoed by Guillemard (1983), who traces the development of contemporary images of ageing and life-styles of older people in France to the shifting debates around retirement and pension provision. However, where Cowgill simply notes industrialisation as one element of modern society, Guillemard demonstrates that its impact on the creation of a specific cultural form of old age is neither fixed or unitary. In particular, Guillemard (1983, pp. 93–4) focuses on the economic and political divisions around which the contemporary identity of old age in France is structured. So for Guillemard the analysis of old age is not only a matter of culture; it is also interwoven with the material aspects of economic and political life. This is not to deny the importance of ideology and culture, or their relative autonomy with respect to the material dimension, but rather to deny a primacy to the ideological sphere which obscures economic and political structures and action, so confusing their connections with culture.

It is important, therefore, in recognising the limitations of the modernisation theory, not to suggest that it has no relevance to debates about ageing and old age in advanced industrial societies. There is undoubtedly continuing change affecting older people as part of wider society. Moreover, the potential advent of the 'post-industrial' and 'post-modern' society appears increasingly to take on a reality and this can be expected to have significant implications for what it means to be an older person (Touraine, 1969; Bell, 1973; Achenbaum and Stearns, 1978; Gruman, 1978; Giddens, 1991). In this sense the questions raised by the modernisation theory about the ideological and cultural *meaning* of old age in contemporary society retain a critical importance, and one to which I will return several times in later chapters. The ideological construction of ageing and old age must also be placed in the relevant historical, economic, political and social context.

Demography

One of the major material factors associated with ageing and old age in contemporary industrial society is that of demographic change. As I have shown above, the demographic approach to old age is centred around the issues of the growth of the numbers of older people, globally as well as in European society, and the relationship this has to other sections of populations (Victor, 1987; de Jouvenal, 1988; Evers and Olk, 1991; Johnson and Falkingham, 1992; Robolis, 1993). The cornerstones of this analysis are fertility rates, mortality rates and the extent of international migration (de Jouvenal, 1988, p. 8). The coming together of these dimensions in advanced industrial societies has meant that three related patterns have emerged: an increase in the proportion of older people in the population; an increase in the actual number of older people; and an increase in the average age of populations (de Jouvenal, 1988, p. 6).

The outcome for Europe is that the proportion of people aged over 65 years is expected to double in the latter half of the twentieth century, while the percentage of people aged over 75 is anticipated to increase by a little under three times (United Nations, 1986). This has led some commentators to talk of 'demographic disaster', or to refer to a 'demographic time bomb'. These concepts anticipate a point in the near future where, if present trends continue, an 'imbalance' of older people to younger people will be reached in so far as the changed proportions will have profound effects on every aspect of social organisation. The 'crisis' or 'time-bomb' ideas are based on an assumed link between the absolute numbers and proportions of older people and the ratio of dependence. This ratio is the number of people economically 'active' compared to those who are in some way economically 'dependent' (such as school or college students, or those in receipt of pensions).

However, the figures which provide the basis for concern about dependency levels also reveal that the dramatic change is not in the overall ratio but in the balance between the so-called dependent groups within it (that is, between younger and older people) (Coleman and Bond, 1990; Pitaud *et al.*, 1991; Johnson and Falkingham, 1992).

Yet, as both de Jouvenal (1988) and Johnson and Falkingham (1992) argue, the idea of crisis arises from presumptions about the dependence (economic and otherwise) of older people which are derived not only from predicted numbers and proportions but also at the same time from particular perceptions of old age as a part of human experience. So the 'demographic crisis' idea is based on particular assumptions about ageing, such as adaptability to change, capacity to develop new skills, or to make an active contribution to society, which are more correctly seen as generational or cohort characteristics rather than the consequences of age *per se*, where they are evident at all (Hendricks and Hendricks, 1977; Gruman, 1978; de Jouvenal, 1988; Evers and Olk, 1991; Johnson and Falkingham, 1992).

The reason why fertility rates are an important aspect of the demographic approach is that the increase in the proportions of older people in European societies does not arise solely from the growth in actual numbers of those aged over 65 years and a decline in mortality rates but also from the decline in the numbers of people aged less than 20 years and of birth-rates. In this sense the concept of an 'ageing' population relates to the age structure of society *as a whole* and not to one segment in isolation. Proportionately fewer people are being born as well as more people living longer. This phenomenon both supports and at the same time casts additional doubt on the veracity of the 'demographic crisis' idea. Although it forms part of the concept of a 'time bomb' in that it suggests that in future years the numbers of economically active adults will decline, this analysis ignores both the consequence that there will be fewer younger dependent people and that the definition of old age in this sense is not fixed. For example, current knowledge about the levels of fertility would allow for the review of the age of retirement (to compensate for a smaller pool of those who economically active) the setting of which is a sociopolitical construction.

Furthermore, current 'time bomb' or 'crisis' concepts fail to take into account other potential changes in economic structures and work patterns such as those arising from technological developments or from changes in the gender structure of the labour market. In their crudest form they extrapolate only the gross population figures (de Jouvenal, 1988, p. 40; Coleman and Bond, 1990, p. 5). As has been noted above, they add to this presuppositions about the capacities of older people, although recent evidence from the UK is that the deliberate employment of older people in retailing can show tangible benefits economically (despite initially being forced on the company concerned because of unusual local circumstances) (Johnson and Falkingham, 1992, p. 182). In short, any 'problem' is not one of older people, but one for all members of society (including the young and the middle-aged) in how different age groups relate economically, politically and culturally. Expressed in these terms it is possible also to reassert that age is only one social dimension, and that gender and sexuality, race and ethnicity, and class are all factors which should be included in any analysis.

It is this question of 'crisis' which demonstrates both the necessity and also the weakness of the demographic approach to ageing. This criticism of the means towards which quantitative analysis is directed does not seek to detract from the importance of being able to delineate accurately the scale of ageing or its relationships to other aspects of society. What it does reveal is that the meaning of the figures remains a matter of interpretation and so requires an underpinning social theory which makes explicit its assumptions. In this sense the demographic approach is a necessary but not a sufficient basis for the development of a *social* gerontology. It cannot explain change but it is essential to describe the complexities of the changes taking place (Tinker, 1981).

Political economy

This theoretical approach begins from the perspective that old age is a social construction and one which must be understood in terms of both its material and ideological dimensions (Guillemard, 1981, 1983; Walker, 1981, 1986b; Phillipson, 1982; Fennell *et al.*, 1988). Drawing explicitly on a materialist understanding of social structures and relationships, this approach stresses the way in which old age in industrial society cannot be understood separately from that society (Bond, 1986). Possibilities for experiencing old age are seen as being created and sustained within the social terrain of industrial capitalism, underpinned by economic relations (Esping-Andersen, 1990). The importance of retirement from paid employment as a boundary marker for old age, for example, then becomes clearly identified (Phillipson, 1982, 1990).

This perspective also provides a very clear analytic basis for examining social divisions within the group defined as older people. The major themes which have been identified have been issues of class and gender, with a critique of conceptions of old age which do not account for such divisions (Walker, 1981, 1990; Phillipson, 1982; Guillemard, 1983). More recently this focus has been broadened to account for the racial, ethnic and cultural divisions of European societies, as well as the developing economic relationships in which patterns of consumption have taken on an increasing significance in considering distinctions between different groups of older people (Bornat *et al.*, 1985; Featherstone and Hepworth, 1986; Fennell *et al.*, 1988).

Nevertheless, these additional dimensions represent a refinement of the political economy approach rather than a departure from it in that they still concern the differential access of distinct social groups to *resources* which provide the basis for living in old age, whether these are economic, political, cultural or social.

The primary focus of this approach on the social construction of old age through exclusion from waged labour has also served to emphasise the *relative* nature of the phenomenon of old age. That is, to the extent that the boundary between middle age and old age is fixed around withdrawal from the labour market, and this in turn is the product of sociopolitical judgements, then old age as a social category is an artefact rather than the elucidation of 'natural' age-related capacities. It is as much the product of the social structures of advanced capitalism as merchandise is the product of a factory, or services are the product of the professions. Moreover, like these other types of product, it is subject to change in relation to economic and social circumstances. Debates about the retirement age are couched in terms of the place of older people in society, not in the abstract as an attempt to locate the 'essence' of old age but in the context of specific questions about the size of the labour force, the costs of retirement and so on.

It is at this juncture that the political economy approach can be regarded as connecting the questions which are posed separately by modernisation theories and demographics, of the ideological and material dimensions of old age. This can be seen in Guillemard's (1983) analysis of older people in France which reintroduced a concern with the sociopolitical 'image of ageing' into this framework. Guillemard (1983, pp. 79 ff.) shows how there have been three periods in the latter half of the twentieth century in France in which there has been a shift in emphasis from the standard of living for older people (access to economic resources) to a concern with way of life and social integration (access to political and cultural resources) and, more recently, indications of a return to standard-of-living issues related to demographic changes within specific economic circumstances.

It is argued that the focus on basic rights of older people to income became displaced by debates on the social meaning of old age as a natural part of the life-cycle (from which the idea of the 'third age' has emerged) only when those rights were secure. Since the late 1970s the economic situation has reintroduced old age as a component in the struggles around industrial and fiscal crises, with the development of concepts such as 'early retirement' or 'pre-retirement redundancy'. In this analysis, both the meaning attached to being older and the realities of ageing populations are brought together.

However, as Guillemard (1983, p. 94) also shows, the return to 'standard of living' questions has occurred in the context of a greater general awareness of old age as 'everyone's future'. The middle classes have expanded throughout the twentieth century, to the point where they have accumulated intellectual and financial resources and aspirations, while the working classes in the later part of this century have come to regard welfare responses as a right rather than as charity. These changes have meant that over only a few decades the cultural models of old age and the policy options which are related to them have shifted dramatically. Struggles over the way of life in the 'third age' are not easily dismissed simply because economic growth has not proved sustainable. Because there are different class groupings within the wider category of 'older people' it must be recognised also that an age-related solidarity as such is unlikely to develop. But nevertheless, perhaps even arising from this social fragmentation, old age has become a politically volatile arena (Bond, 1986). For this reason a 'redenigration' of need in older age as a policy option to support reduced levels of public welfare, including the provision of public pension schemes, is not necessarily an easy alternative (Groves, 1987; Dieck, 1990). This conclusion serves to underline the extent to which the organisation and experience of old age is contextualised within the economic, political and cultural circumstances of a particular place and time. (Historical and anthropological perspectives will be discussed further in Chapters 2 and 3.)

Conceptual conflict or complementarity?

It is not my intention here simply to catalogue three major theoretical approaches, but rather to address the implications that they have for the study of old age and so for the discussions which follow. I am beginning from the position that any analysis necessarily involves a theoretical standpoint, whether this is implicit or explicit, and that conscious theorising in gerontology is both necessary and desirable (Myles, 1983; Fennell *et al.*, 1988). In this I am following the mid-range applied perspective of Fennell *et al.*, rather than the more abstract sociological framework outlined by Myles (although some sociological concepts do lie behind the mid-range). This perspective owes something to Mills' (1970) injunction to be flexible between theoretical and empirical aspects of study, so that the discussion can be focused on a range of phenomena (historical, cultural, social and so on). For this reason also, much of the more detailed conceptual work which has been developed, such as Victor's (1987) delineation of 'approaches' to the study of ageing (social problems, disengagement, symbolic interaction, activity, labelling and stratification), should be seen to be of a secondary order (as very specific conceptual positions). These issues will be introduced in the following chapters at the points where they are relevant. However, they are also derived from more general social theory and it is necessary first to clarify the balance between material and ideological explanations of social structures and processes which underpin more particular enquiries. Modernisation theory (with a focus on the ideological construction of old age), demography of old age (grounded in an empirical focus on material aspects of ageing), and political economy of old age (which begins from a material standpoint while seeking to relate this to ideological structures) represent more basic examples of the way in which social theories create particular understandings of ageing and the construction of old age.

Yet are these theoretical approaches to be seen as conflicting and competing, or is there an extent to which they are complementary? At face value it may seem that the modernisation thesis and demographics are seeking to answer different types of question about old age: the former about changes in the meaning attached to old age in modern society while the latter concerns the statistical profile of older age within the overall population, such that they might be complementary. As we have seen above, it is not possible to consider the meaning of old age without looking at the scale and location of older people within the wider society. Conversely, empirical facts do not speak for themselves and the explanation of statistical changes necessitate presumptions about the experience and meaning of old age. In either case, the extent to which all aspects of ageing and old age as social phenomena can be encompassed is limited. However, neither perspective appears to have sought integration with the other and although each makes use of insights which belong within the other frame of reference, there is no explicit synthesis or connection.

The analysis of the political economy approach to social gerontology has sought to extend the scope of enquiry in just this way, bringing together ideological and material facets of ageing. This synthesis has enabled the perspective to recognise that old age is a social phenomenon, that it is contested and so is political (in the broadest sense) (Estes, 1979; Guillemard, 1983; Kart, 1987; Phillipson and Walker, 1987). Bond (1986) argues that some critics of the political economy perspective have discounted it because of what is seen as an overtly neo-Fabian or neo-Marxist orientation (irrespective of the explicit political stance of such critics), although this is not necessarily the case. However, the identification of the origins of the contemporary experience and meaning of old age in the structures and relationships of capitalist industrial society, particularly the inequalities and dependencies of old age, is likely to be contested ground (Guillemard, 1983; Walker, 1981, 1986b). Moreover, in so far as all study embodies social theory, this is unlikely to be separable from debates about wider social structures and relationships, whether these concern the family, health and welfare, or the nature of old age (George and Wilding, 1976; Offe, 1984; Bornat *et al.*, 1985).

The emergence of political economy as a major theoretical approach, if not a dominant perspective, may be regarded as a consequence of its attention not to the material facts of old age or to the ideological meaning surrounding the phenomenon in isolation from each other, but to the connections between the two. This is not to say that pertinent questions are not raised by the other two approaches which have been discussed, and some aspects of these are examined in the following chapters. What will be clear in the way the discussion unfolds, however, is that this book is based on the premise that ageing and old age are social constructions and does not seek to test this assumption as such but rather to explore the implications that it brings to understanding the phenomenon of old age in Europe. In this sense the empirical facts and the meaning of ageing are contextualised within a wider understanding of European social structures and relationships, which provides the basis for identifying specific topics for scrutiny, such as the family, industrial and economic relations, religion, welfare policies and practices and so on.

The Focus of this Book

A comparative approach to ageing

I have referred above to the rapid change which is taking place in the shape of Europe. Not only is Europe undergoing economic and political transformation, but this is occurring against a background of historical and cultural diversity. In looking at ageing and old age in this context it is necessary for this diversity to be acknowledged and addressed. It is not possible to discuss Europe as a single entity at more than the broadest level. For that reason Chapter 2 begins with an exploration of the comparative analysis of old age, considering key examples in anthropological, historical and sociological studies. This is intended both to provide the foundation for the approach which will follow and to begin to sketch out some of the issues which can be seen in the recognition of old age as a relative social phenomenon.

Following from this discussion of comparative method, an illustrative model juxtaposing two countries will be developed in the second part of Chapter 2, both to consider the possibilities and limitations of this approach and to establish a model for the wider consideration of the broader range of European countries which forms the content of Chapter 3. Chapter 2 will also be the base for the structure of the remainder of the book, where the themes for subsequent discussion are identified.

Focus on social responses to ageing

The overall focus of this book is on the relationship between material circumstances, the meaning of old age in European society, and forms of social response to ageing. Such a focus takes the discussion through a model of factors affecting perceptions of old age to a consideration of the concrete forms of health and welfare policies and practices which have developed to meet the perceived needs of older people.

This focus is adopted because old age as a 'social issue' centres on the perceived connection between ageing and the implications of changes in the older populations of European countries which have been noted above. This is not to say that old age is synonymous with dependence, or necessarily to talk of older people in the passive voice (Fennell *et al.*, 1988, pp. 6–8). Both these points are topics for investigation (and to which I will return at several places in the following chapters).

To return to an objection which I noted above, Fennell *et al.* (1988), following Johnson (1976), argue that the close connection between ageing and social need in gerontological study leads to a 'pathologising' of old age and older people. That is, as a stage in the human life-course, later years become typified as 'abnormal' and 'problematic' and are therefore ascribed negative connotations, even though the demographic data demonstrate that it is now 'normal' for people in Europe to live beyond the age of 70 years (see p. 7). This objection does not deny that for some older people the latter part of their life is experienced as problematic, because of low income, poor housing, limited access to a wide social life, and particular difficulties in health and welfare. Rather, as we have seen, it suggests that these problems arise from the social organisation of responses to old age rather than from the nature of ageing itself. So it is important to acknowledge that for many older people life is indeed full of potential and opportunity.

At the same time, however, a critical social gerontology cannot ignore the issues surrounding the structural inequalities which are part of the social construction of old age, and which are translated into perceptions of need and from there into health and welfare responses. Older people who are not 'in need' (those people who are wealthy, healthy and so on) are still to an extent incorporated within this process, in so far as it feeds back into the related phenomenon of ageism, that is, the irrelevant discrimination between people on grounds of age (which will be discussed in greater detail in Chapter 4) (Gruman, 1978; Itzin, 1986). But then, it could be asked whether there are any grounds for talking about older people separately from other social groups, apart from the extent to which the issues they face are socially constructed around biological age. Otherwise, should our attention not be focused on the wider groups of men and women, white and black, heterosexual and homosexual, disabled and non-disabled, rich and poor, or (to pursue another angle) of those who are interested in opera, dog-racing, knitting or hang-gliding?

So this book is not only concerned with ageing and old age as such, but also with the framework of social responses to these phenomena, especially as these have been expressed as 'caring' about and for older people in its broadest sense through health and welfare in different European countries (Ungerson, 1983; Hugman, 1991). This book is about ageing in relation to the social welfare responses to old age. In the next chapter I will map out the comparative background to this approach and establish the model which will be developed in the following chapters, leading towards a consideration of the contemporary issues facing European society in relation to older people.

2

Polarities and Similarities: An Outline Framework

Comparative Approaches

The cross-national comparative study of old age

It is only in recent times that a concern with the global range of human experience in ageing has become identified as an issue for study in gerontology (Palmore, 1980, p. xvii). This phenomenon is in itself instructive, in that the concentration of gerontological study in North America and Northern Europe is a reflection of underlying social processes. As we shall see, these have brought together the increased longevity and greater proportions of populations defined as 'elderly' with particular welfare responses and the interest of professionals and academics to understand and respond to ageing. As a consequence, comparative work, even recently, has been centred around the perspectives of the dominant societies that have been labelled as the 'First World', although there have been some interesting contributions from social anthropology (Cowgill, 1972; Palmore, 1980; Victor, 1987; Fennell *et al.*, 1988). So to propose the construction of a single comparative method is both premature and unhelpful. More relevant is a critical review of the diversity of approaches which have been taken to the comparative study of ageing and old age.

The work of Shanas *et al.* (1968) may be regarded as the classic cross-national sociological study of old age. It examines three countries: Denmark, Great Britain and the United States. The authors' objective was to develop an understanding of the way in which cultural and socio-structural differences affected the conditions and conduct of older people, focusing especially on the concept of 'disengagement' (Shanas *et al.*, 1968, p. 3). They concluded that it is not a functional feature of old age as a social role (as had been claimed by Cumming and Henry, 1961), but the

21

consequence of social forces which keep *some* older people integrated yet marginalise others as well as stigmatising 'old age' as a phenomenon (Shanas *et al.*, 1968, p. 425). At the same time as this general conclusion was reached, it was noted also that there are differences between the three countries studied, which suggests that economic, political and social structures do have an impact on the construction and experience of old age (Shanas *et al.*, pp. 424 ff.).

The major strength of this study lies in its comparative method. Whereas previous work had relied on material accumulated in different ways and in response to different problems, Shanas *et al.* (1968, p. 3, pp. 13–14) asked the same questions in each country (allowing for translation), which were based on the same research problematic, namely whether old age in industrial society is to be understood in relation to integration and disengagement. Its major weakness lies in the scale, which enables authoritative statements to be made on a relatively general level but which may serve to obscure more specific but nevertheless useful and interesting points (Fennell *et al.*, 1988, p. 74).

Shanas *et al.* (1968, p. 14) are clear that, in their view, adequate comparative study is dependent on methodological rigour of the type which can only be achieved in a single controlled project; all else, they argue, is trivial. However, while I would not wish to dispute the underlying methodological point, that the collection of data may set limits on the uses to which they can be put, this appears to restrict the possibility of cross-national investigation to large-scale empirical surveys. Comparing 'like with like' gives greater control over objectivity, but where the data to which we have access are not alike, then it may be sufficient to be aware of how they differ and to incorporate this awareness into any analysis. This is not the same as the production of trivia.

In the anthropological field a major comparative analysis has been undertaken by Silverman and Maxwell (1982). They say that relatively little attention appears to have been paid by anthropologists to the topic of ageing and older people, suggesting a marginalisation of this issue from that discipline until anthropologists brought it all back home in the form of urban ethnography (Silverman and Maxwell, 1982, pp. 46–7). (The work of Cowgill and Holmes (1972) and de Beauvoir's (1977) summary of ethnological data perhaps set the boundaries to this claim as they point also to earlier studies.) Silverman and Maxwell (1982, pp. 62–7) analysed data from ninety-six societies, noting the wide variation of cultural perspectives concerning the social position and role of older people. Their conclusions are broad, but provide a basis for further empirical examination. Ageing, they argue, is a positive part of social life if older people are socially active, occupying non-trivial roles linked to strong community boundaries and clear social structures. In particular, control by older people over information and resources (whether material or symbolic) are important. Silverman and Maxwell also conclude that ageing is gendered almost universally, with power and esteem clearly divided patriarchally in all the societies they considered. In short, that old men fare better than old women appears to be a rare example of an anthropological absolute.

Victor (1987, pp. 76–84) also provides a comparative resumé of anthropological work, noting the wide diversity of responses to old age that have been observed in 'preindustrial' societies. This comparison of case material provides an insight into anthropology, in that most of the studies quoted view responses to old age in starkly positive or negative terms; there seems little room for ambiguity. From Victor's comparative discussion, a more detailed conclusion emerges, noting that the position of older people in these societies was structured around certain key issues:

1. The type of social organisation (such as nomadic or settled);
2. The physical status of the older person (for example, frailty);
3. The social importance of the experience of older people;
4. The economic or cultural value of the activity of older people;
5. The extent of control by older people over knowledge, ritual or religious practice;
6. The extent to which older people maintain the status of activity from which they have now retired; and
7. The extent of control by older people over others through control of scarce resources or political power (Victor, 1987, pp. 83–4).

Each of these factors, it is argued, is a necessary but not sufficient explanation of the situation of older people in any given society. Possibly the only anthropological absolute in this context appears to be the categorisation of part of the life-cycle as 'old age' in all known societies.

In addition, both Silverman and Maxwell (1982) and Victor (1987) identify certain themes which are useful for the study of contemporary Europe, including the occurrence of what may be seen as ill-treatment and neglect rather than veneration of older people, and the extent to which some concept of kinship obligation for the care of dependent older people is widespread.

The earlier work of Stearns (1977) and that of Minois (1989) together represent a different approach to ageing and old age in Europe, taking an historical perspective in both cases. This approach is claimed by Stearns to have originated as recently as the mid-1970s (Stearns, 1977, p. 13). Both studies are comparative. Stearns' detailed analysis of France is set within an understanding of the broader European context, while Minois' (1989) discussion is wide-ranging, spanning more than two millenia and several cultures and countries. The underlying implication, which may be drawn from the chronological panorama developed by the historical approach, is that 'old age' as a social concept has had a history as well as a geography, developing differently in diverse contexts but nevertheless changing markedly over time. It has been argued that from the ancient Middle East, to the early Middle Ages in Europe, to recent non-industrial Africa, old age has often been associated with the qualitative accumulation of experience. In contrast, modern industrial European constructions are based on the quantitative accumulation of physical years (Gruman, 1978; Minois, 1989).

Yet it is possible to idealise the understanding of and social attitudes to old age in other times or places: the *mythos* of the 'Golden Age' (Stearns, 1977, p. 11). Evidence of the misery of elderly people (for example, because of poverty or ill health), or the actual denigration of older people despite formal ideologies of veneration, can be seen in historical as well as anthropological data (Fennell *et al.*, 1988; Minois, 1989). What we find, most frequently, is an ambivalence or even ambiguity about old age and elderly people which at best sets some negative aspects of reality against the positive images and often undermines that which might be positive. The value of ageing may be conditional on other factors being met (health, knowledge, wealth and so on) and so may only be open to some older people, while others are regarded as a burden or expendable. Considering old age across time as well as space reinforces the caution which one should exercise in over-generalising rosy pictures that perhaps say more about ideology in the contemporary situation than they do about other epochs or places.

A number of themes run through these comparative studies, whether contemporary or historical, in that together they point to the structuring of old age on a range of dimensions, including political structures, economic factors, industrialisation and urbanisation, gender divisions and the family, health and hygiene, ideological constructions (such as honour or esteem) and professional and political responses to older people. Each of these is also bound up with the respective cultures of periods and places. In summary, old age is a socially and culturally relative phenomenon.

More recently a number of studies have sought to provide a range of data without developing the necessary integrating framework which can be said to provide the comparative dimension (Warnes, 1987a). Teicher *et al.* (1979), Palmore (1980), Evers and Svetlik (1991) and Kraan *et al.* (1991) make available a diversity of data which is both useful and necessary in the

the most truly comparative analysis is to be found in the middle of the range; that which is focused on a specified set of countries, and asking the same questions of each.

For the reasons outlined above, however, I will not be seeking to construct a typological comparative framework in the manner of Little (1979) or Kosberg (1992) in the following chapters. Nor do I want simply to extend the use of Titmuss's welfare-state model. Rather, I am concerned to examine the range of factors which may be used to identify and extend a theoretical understanding of ageing in European societies. There are weaknesses also in this approach to comparative work in that it does require the use of data which will have been recorded for a variety of purposes. As a consequence, the outcome may at times have a 'patchwork' quality in which it is not possible for the range of countries discussed to be treated equally. In order to establish a conceptual framework from which to begin, the second part of this chapter will explore a comparison between two countries as the basis for the subsequent wider discussion of ageing and older people across Europe.

The uses of comparative work

The comparative study of old age and elderly people serves two purposes: the first is to develop a broader understanding of the social processes in question; and the second to learn about and develop new ways of responding to the interests and needs of older people. I am concerned here with both aspects.

In the previous section of this chapter I outlined briefly the way in which cross-national, cross-cultural or historical studies can lead to a fuller understanding of this topic. A diversity of information and interpretation can enable greater exactitude in the analysis of particular instances (Stearns, 1977; Jones, 1985). Yet this is not the whole story, in that it is difficult, if not impossible, to divorce an interest in knowing *about* from a concern with knowing *for*. By this I mean that we cannot divorce the policy implications of the apparently recent surge in gerontological work, much of which is hedged around with questions about the rapid increase in numbers of elderly people in industrial society, from more theoretical concerns about ageing and developing responses to perceived needs of older people (Havighurst, 1978; Gilleard *et al.*, 1985). Terms such as 'challenge' or even 'anxiety' and 'alarm' have been used, although these can be opposed by the more positive 'grey revolution' or a concern to identify and contest 'ageism' (Gaullier, 1982; Bornat *et al.*, 1985; Noin and Warnes, 1987). We want to know not just so that we can know, but also so that we can do something. Our knowledge is tied to the objective of developing more insightful responses to old age and elderly people which might be congruent with the social values to which we aspire.

Here I agree with Fennell *et al.* (1988, p. 6) when they observe that to 'take a benign interest in other's problems' involves a number of risks, of which the first is that we 'welfarise' the subject of our study, and that we learn to meet need rather than to understand the causes of that need. It is the former perspective (knowledge directed *only* to meeting need), despite good intentions, which does much to pathologise old age. However, provided the distinction is recognised, and each perspective is allowed its legitimate sphere, there is a danger also in forgetting about the purposes of knowledge (Barnes, 1979). Even if it is the case that most elderly people do not have dependency needs beyond the range of human needs usually observed in younger adults, we should be concerned both with helping people to avoid dependency where this is not necessary (especially where dependency results from misunderstanding) and providing the best possible responses when they are required. It is in this sense that comparative study is a useful ground for knowledge which is valid in scientific terms but is also capable of being applied. The transfer of learning between various national contexts provides a basis for being more critical in our approach, towards both knowledge and policy.

The basis of a comparison within Europe

The focus of this book is Europe, and especially those countries which comprise the European Community. The basis of comparison here is one which may be said to be marked more by diversity than by a uniform heritage. To some degree there is a sense of shared history, of cultural origins in the common well of ancient Greece and Rome, and of Judaeo-Christian traditions. Europe has an identity separate from that of Africa, Asia, the Americas or Australasia (even though in recent centuries its culture has been exported on a global basis, and aspects of other cultures absorbed) (Brittan and Maynard, 1984).

At the same time, within the recognition of these limits, there is a wide diversity which, as we will see, plays a part in understanding the development of old age and responses to older people in the different European countries (Haller, 1990). Celtic, Teutonic, Anglo-Saxon, Scandinavian, Hispanic, Slavonic, Latin and Greek cultural influences have shaped European history, so that dividing Europe north/south, or east/west, or by even finer distinctions, shapes the conclusions at which one could arrive. Similarly, in the question of religion, although Europe may be said to have been predominantly Christian for more than 1500 years, this religion has three major subdivisions in the continent, namely Orthodox, Roman Catholic and Protestant. These three groups have each been influential in different parts of Europe, in relation to other social phenomena such as the family and the economy, and in that sense their pattern of dispersal is a crucial marker to the variety within an apparent uniformity (see also Tawney, 1926; Weber, 1930).

In the contemporary era the nation states of Europe are divided not only by cultural background and religion, but also by economic and political development and structures. (I will return below to the question of how these might be related.) As we have seen, the studies of older people by Shanas *et al.* (1968), Stearns (1977), Little (1979), Minois (1989) and Kosberg (1992) among others have demonstrated the centrality of these issues for a consideration of older people and the social responses to them.

It is on the basis of differences in these respects that I have selected two nation states, Greece and the UK, as the illustration for an outline construction of a comparative framework. These two countries may be regarded as being at 'opposite ends' of the EC, socially as well as geographically. Not only are they located physically in the south-east and north-west of the EC respectively, with the attendant variation in geology and climate, but they are also polarised on a social continuum.

These differences can be seen, for example, in the degree and extent of industrialisation, which in the UK may be traced back to the seventeenth and eighteenth centuries, while in Greece is a twentieth-century phenomenon (Pantelouris, 1987; Petmesidou and Tsoulouvis, 1991), or they may be seen in political history, as Greece in its present form has existed only since 1947 having achieved some initial independence from colonial rule in 1827, whereas the UK has existed since 1800, contracting to its present form in 1921 (Clogg, 1986; Hoppen, 1989). More centrally to the topic of this book, although they have similar proportions of elderly people in their populations – in 1985 slightly more than 11 per cent of the populations of both were aged over 65 years (Pantelouris, 1987, p. 131; Jefferys and Thane, 1989, p. 7) – the demographic changes of Greece have been much more rapid in the second half of the twentieth century, while the demographic 'ageing' of the UK has developed more gradually since the nineteenth century. (I will return below to the point that the 'ageing' of the population is related to a decline in the birth-rate as well as to greater longevity, and in Greece also to emigration; see, for example, Dontas, 1987, and Pantelouris, 1987).

In addition, the two countries have divergent forms of welfare provision. In the UK there has been an extensive welfare state since 1948, but in

Greece welfare state developments may be regarded as being much more limited (Zarras, 1980; Thane, 1982; Stathopoulos and Amera, 1992). This aspect of comparison is of particular importance in considering older people, who are the major users of health care provision in industrialised countries (Warnes, 1987a; Dontas *et al.*, 1991).

In the remainder of this chapter I will examine the ways in which these aspects of social structure may be used to form a comparative understanding of old age in these two countries, and in the following chapters to develop a framework for a broader analysis across Europe.

History and Culture

Political development

Greece may be regarded as having a considerably more ancient identity than the UK, and its culture is rich with images of ageing, albeit very ambivalent (Minois, 1989; Featherstone and Hepworth, 1990). For example, despite an abiding popular conception of the government of ancient Greece resting in the hands of a gerontocracy, Minois warns against overgeneralisation, noting that in the earlier classical periods elderly people were frequently ridiculed and excluded from public life, and that it was only in later peroids, when Greece became more open to foreign influences, that old age was less stigmatised (Minois, 1989, pp. 75–6). The concept of 'elder' (*geras*) referred to honour and reward, usually accorded to exploits in battle, rather than chronological age (a point noted above in relation to other cultures and periods). What Minois does not specify, but which is clear from his account, is that the Greek polity was starkly divided on grounds of gender and class; the elders were all men of the dominant class, so the idea of gerontocracy (literally, rule by old men) is mistaken only in so far as the relationship between 'the old' and 'the elder' is misunderstood. A more recent, nineteenth-century example from the island of Chios, in which elders from the indigenous aristocracy acted as *de facto* governors on behalf of the Ottoman rulers, is given by Clogg (1976, pp. 13–14). These elders were chosen on the basis of wealth and civic distinction rather than age.

This cultural influence on ideologies of the role of older people in political life appears to have survived the following millenium, in which Greece declined and the UK was created. The idea of the elder as the natural repository of political authority drew heavily on themes from ancient European culture. However, it has been argued that although the classicalism of the education system in the UK (especially of the nineteenth and early twentieth centuries) stressed the influence of Greek and Latin ideas in Europe, in this context such a view may be regarded as a distortion because evidence of the veneration of older people comes rather from Anglo-Saxon writings (Burrow, 1986). Here, again, it is essential to be aware of the distinction between 'older' and 'elder', and Minois (1989, p. 141) suggests that old men in Anglo-Saxon society could in some ways be seen as lacking authority. While it seems apparent that, in contrast to ancient Greece, there was more of an association between age and social status in Anglo-Saxon society, the polity was linked as much to other factors (for example, wealth or military power) and the respect accorded to age *per se* was still somewhat diffuse.

In addition to ideologies concerning the political involvement of older people, the histories of these two countries are marked also by significant differences in respect of the impact of wider political structures and events on old age in their societies. An important aspect of these structures is independence, as this has affected the types of political development which have taken place, as well as the opportunity for external influences to play a part in the social construction of ageing. As I noted above, whereas the UK has been a colonial power for more than three hundred years, Greece was colonised for considerably longer, by the Italians, by the Turks and by the British. Indeed, the UK as an entity emerged from the widening power of a strong central monarchy which had grown over the preceding six hundred years, partly by conquest and colonisation. As such, both the opportunity for the shaping of social policy, including that concerned with 'old age' has had a more continuous development than in Greece, and this can be seen most clearly in the foundations of the welfare state which may be traced back to the Elizabethan Poor Law (Thane, 1982). Greece re-emerged into independence only during the last hundred and fifty years, without any such foundations in place.

A further factor in this period of recent Greek history has been the emigration and internal migration of younger people in response to social changes in rural areas (Dontas, 1987; Sant Cassia, 1992). Before 1912 most emigration was to the USA, and later in the twentieth century this broadened to include Western Europe, Canada and Australia. Internally, the same time period saw a large movement of younger people to the towns. This had two effects: the 'ageing' of the population as a whole; and, the reduction in family size in the urban centres. Both factors have contributed to the rapid demographic shifts which were evident in Northern Europe in earlier periods.

Indeed, the starkness of the political dimension to the comparison also may be continued into the twentieth century. It was between 1912 and 1922 that the major part of modern Greece was brought together in independence. The migration from Asia Minor in 1922 brought in about 1.5 million refugees to a country with a population at the time of only 4.5 million; these refugees were settled in just a few months and included a relatively large proportion of older people (Dontas, 1987). It was only in 1947 that the final parts of modern Greece, the Dodecanese Islands, were incorporated in the nation state (Clogg, 1986). At the same time the structures of the modern welfare state in the UK were being transformed in the creation of the national health service and other post-war welfare developments (Thane, 1982).

The subsequent political period in the UK has seen a shift recently in the impact of New Right conservatism on welfare (to which I will return below), but can be said to have been remarkably calm compared to the swing from liberal democracy to dictatorship (in the Colonels' junta of 1967–74) and back again that has occurred in Greece (Clogg, 1986; Pantelouris, 1987). In the UK, policies towards elderly people have been much higher on the political agenda than in Greece, where other issues have held sway.

The implications of this comparison define the first set of boundaries which I want to consider as part of a comparative framework: that political history plays a part in defining how older people are perceived, and the type of services which are offered to them. Here it is suggested that the developing form of political structure, understood as part of the modern historical process, shapes the ground for possible state responses to older people. Ancient history, however, appears to provide an ideological reference point while having little impact in the face of contemporary issues.

Social history and religion

In some senses it may be said that the colonisation of Greece by other countries and the colonisation of other countries by the UK have both served to create a diversity of social relationships which affect older people through the impact on cultural forms, especially of the family or religion. Experiences of colonialism in Greece and the UK appear to have been markedly different. Yet have they necessarily been affected in diametrically opposing ways in relation to cultural forms? In part, both countries may be said to have multicultural influences shaping their contemporary patterns of life, while both arrived in the present era from a dominant religious background of Christianity. However, there are also several differences. First, Greek culture has absorbed influences from others, especially Turkish, from the perspective of the colonised. This is assimilation by the powerless on the terms of the powerful. In contrast, the UK, itself a multi-cultural construction in which at an earlier stage the Anglo-Saxon both dominated and absorbed the Celtic, has continued to assimilate other cultural influences, largely on the terms of the indigenous majority. It has been the colonial centre, bringing home the fruits of colonialism. Greek culture, and the place of old age within it, has been reasserted in the context of recently gained nationhood, often consciously recalling the past. In contrast, that of the UK has been modified by the partial and uneasy assim-ilations of post-colonialism, in which there is a more ambiguous relation-ship with the past as well as present influences from post-colonial settlers (Williamson and Pampel, 1991). This may be seen, for example, in the ambivalence afforded in white UK society to the place of elderly people in black and Asian cultures (Bhalla and Blakemore, 1981; Norman, 1985).

Possibly the most central aspect of culture to affect social responses to ageing and elderly people has been religion, both because of the broad anthropological presuppositions which are contained in religious thought and also because of the powerful influence religion has exerted on the structure of family relationships (Sant Cassia, 1992). Greece, still a major centre of Orthodox Christianity, and the UK, a part of the world in which the Protestant break with Roman Catholic Christianity was first made, also are clearly distinct in this respect. While both reflect the earlier concern with *charitas* shown towards those members of society who are not able to care for themselves, or to be cared for by their family, or who do not have a family (for example, in the fifth commandment, 'honour your father and your mother' (Exodus, 20, xii) which had a general intergenerational significance not confined to biological parents or the New Testament refer-ence to 'widows and orphans' (James, 1, xxvii)), other social and political changes have interacted with the religious sentiment to produce modifica-tions. In the history of the UK, as in other north European countries, the growth of Protestantism has been linked to the rise of capitalism (Tawney, 1926; Weber, 1930). Through a theological as well as a philosophical indi-vidualism, *charitas* has become *charity*, weakening the shared, social dimension of this moral principle and replacing it with the more abstract and impersonal duty of the fellow citizen (Smith, 1982).

For example, the Greek Orthodox Church in recent decades has become a major provider of services for older people who have need of social care, in a way which was replicated by the Anglican Church in the nineteenth century but which has subsequently declined (Parry and Parry, 1979; Zarras, 1980; Dontas, 1987; Amira, 1990). However, the creation of modern welfare services and professions in the UK can, in part, be traced back to just such developments. Early social work, nursing and some medical innovations were motivated by religious concern, but mediated through secularisation these areas of social action have been incorporated in the state (Parry and Parry, 1979; Hugman, 1991). In Greece the same separation of political and religious life has not occurred, although there are indications of increasing state intervention in policy responses to the needs of older people (Zarras, 1980; Teperoglou *et al.*, 1990). Yet the church continues to play a major role, in part because it was regarded as a major bastion of Greek culture during centuries of foreign domination (despite controversy over the actual role played by parts of the church hierarchy at specific times), and also because of its established status in the modern state (Clogg, 1976, pp. 107–11; 1986, pp. 23–6; Pantelouris, 1987, p. 138).

Further aspects of social development have been changes in the structure of the family. Well into the twentieth century in Greek society it was the role of older people in the family to exercise authority through the patriarchal control by older men over finances and relationships (such as the marriage of children or grandchildren), and by women over the running of the home. This was organised in a pattern of extended families which survived in some form until relatively recently. The more recent growth of the nuclear family is therefore regarded as weakening more generally the position of older people in society (Psychogios, 1987; Teperoglou *et al.*, 1990; Sant Cassia, 1992). In the UK, in contrast, the nuclear family appears to predate the Industrial Revolution, and it is questionable whether it has ever been common for extended families to be co-resident (Anderson, 1971). The extended families 'discovered' in East London by Willmott and Young (1962) were, it has been argued, the creation of urbanisation, replacing the wider and more diffuse social networks of rural society (Laslett, 1977). Research in some other countries (to which I will return in later chapters) has shown that in urban society family relationships with older members have not necessarily weakened, but rather have become more geographically dispersed (Rosenmayr and Köckeis, 1963). The main change in recent years has not been one of family structure, therefore, but has been associated with greater mobility, especially among middle-class and skilled working-class groups in both Greece and the UK.

In common with Greece, family relationships in the UK have long been patriarchal, although the manner of exercising patriarchal authority has been shaped by its context. The role of the grandparent (and notably the authority of the grandfather) has never been as so great in the UK as in Greece. The place of elderly people within families in the UK can therefore be said to be defined not so much by a weakening as by an adapting role, whereas the weakening role of the Greek grandfather in particular is related also to the modern shape of patriarchal social structures.

In summary it may be noted that the wider social aspects in the history of ageing and the role of elderly people in Greece and the UK differ in respect of their experience of national identity, religion and the family. Indeed, the way in which the traditional nature of Greek society, with a strong central role for older people (especially men) and the strength of traditional religion underpins the Greek struggle for cultural identity is opposed in many ways to the history of the UK in the same period (Clogg, 1976).

Industrialisation

Reference has been made above to the connections identified between religious change and the Industrial Revolution. The Weberian explanation of the links between Protestant Christianity (or, more specifically, its puritan strand) and capitalism has been the subject of extensive debate between sociologists and historians (Bendix, 1966; Eldridge, 1971). However, the central concept, that changes in material relationships and social ideas are interconnected, does suggest that the individualism in Protestant theology and the developing capitalist industrial society on the one hand and corporatism in Orthodox theology and agrarian Mediterranean society on the other are associated to a substantial degree.

The social consequences arising from industrialisation go beyond forms of production which affected the relationship of workers both to their work and to each other as factory systems became predominant, and which also affected family relationships in so far as the home ceased to be the locus of craft work (Briggs, 1968; Braverman, 1974). There is much evidence to suggest that in the urban industrial society of the UK in the nineteenth century older people were no more and no less marginalised than they had been in previous rural life. However, their position was largely related to their capacity to work or to make some other contribution to the domestic economy, or the ownership of property, if they were to have independence and dignity (Quadagno, 1982; Smith, 1982; Phillipson, 1990). This can be seen in the contemporaneous literature of George Eliot, Charles Dickens and Thomas Hardy, among others.

What was seen, however, was a sharper division between the poor older person and those with either wealth or savings. Moreover, the demands for greater efficiency in factory production and government administration led to a greater questioning about the place of older people in the factory or the office (Thane, 1983). The implications this carried for the creation of more large-scale poverty among elderly people became the background for the wider introduction of pensions, and with that institutionalised in the UK in the early part of the twentieth century, the idea of a 'retirement age'

(Phillipson, 1990, p. 146). Variations in the practice of retirement have tended to be in response to economic factors, redefining older people according to the perceived needs of industry for a workforce, rather than in relation to any attributes of older people themselves (Parker, 1982).

In contrast to the UK, Greece has until very recently been an agrarian society (Clogg, 1986; Pantelouris, 1987). The impact of the Industrial Revolution has come to Greece in the latter part of the twentieth century, following political unification. Within the rural society of Greece the place of the older person is often referred to in positive terms (Teperoglou *et al.*, 1990; Stathopoulos and Amera, 1992), and yet there is little to suggest that it was markedly different from the life of older people in the pre-industrial UK. In other words, if the older person had good health (and so could continue to work), or had wealth, then their position would be secured. Otherwise they were dependent on the younger members of their family, without whom they would be the subjects of religious charity. Pensions, of which I will say more in the next section of this chapter, have been a relatively recent phenomenon (Teperoglou *et al.*, 1990).

Recent industrialisation and emigration from Greece has left rural areas with relatively large proportions of older people, while the populations of Athens and Thessaloniki have mushroomed in a manner similar to London, Birmingham, Leeds or Glasgow in the late eighteenth and the nineteenth centuries (Briggs, 1968; Pantelouris, 1987). Although many retired people have followed younger relatives into the cities, many have stayed in the villages and some have returned (Zarras, 1980; Stathopoulos and Amera, 1992). Because this process is more recent in origin than in the UK the proportional balance of younger and older adults in rural areas has changed more rapidly in the twentieth century in Greece.

In this respect the process of urbanisation in Greece appears to be following a similar course to that which has taken place in the UK over the eighteenth and nineteenth centuries. However, it would not be an adequate explanation simply to suggest that Greece is 'following' the UK in an inevitable historical process. As we have seen above, there are been many aspects in which Greece is and has been very different. Nevertheless, this degree of similarity does provide the basis for addressing the possibility that industrialisation, urbanisation and the place of elderly people in society do have some generalisable connections.

Some general points

The histories of Greece and the UK indicate that different social and cultural patterns of development are associated with aspects of constructions of ageing and responses to older people. I have sketched out the relevance of political and economic change, religious thought and urbanisation, with the family appearing as a central focus for the social care of older people who are perceived to be dependent. So, it is to the family that I will turn first in considering some comparisons of the situation of older people in the present day.

Contemporary Social Structures

The family

As we have already seen, there are suggestions that the place of elderly people within the family has been subject to wide-ranging and negative changes. In the UK, for example, recent government policies have been structured around this assumption (Department of Health and Social Security, 1982). This has been so despite considerable research evidence to the contrary (Wenger, 1984; Ungerson, 1987; Hicks, 1988; Finch, 1989; Parker, 1990). In Greece the same negative view of changed roles for elderly people within the family can be seen, and there does appear to be some evidence to support such a view (Zarras, 1980; Psychogios, 1987, Teperoglou *et al.*, 1990; Stathopoulos and Amera, 1992). Berger (1979) identifies within the social process of 'modernity' (as a general phenomenon) a movement from social *roles* to social *relationships* as the defining characteristics of the family. In other words, that the rigid and formal expectations of tradition are replaced by a continually negotiated order, in which reference is made to a wide range of potential influences on what is appropriate or acceptable. As we have seen above, there are often a number of myths attached to this perspective, particularly in the UK, but the concept does recognise the greater fluidity of modern society.

So where do older people fit into the contemporary family? First, as we have already seen, in both Greece and the UK there is diversity in how far older people live from younger family members. Those who live with off-spring are a minority of less than 20 per cent in both countries, even though there may be a formal ideological expression of the desirability of co-residence (some research suggests the Greek proportion may be slightly higher) (Green, 1988; Teperoglou, 1990; Triantafillou and Mestheneos, 1990). For example, the negative views of older people as patients, which are held by some doctors in Athens, are contrasted with strong expressions of warmth from families towards their own co-resident elderly parents (Triantafillou and Mestheneos, 1990).

Occupationally related mobility, especially in the middle classes and skilled working classes, has been a major factor in whether older people are living close to or at a distance from their offspring (Bond, 1990). In the UK there is some mobility among older people themselves, and in the south-east of England it is possible to identify 'retirement counties' which have a net gain of people moving to these on retirement (see, for example, Warnes, 1987b). However, this may be mitigated by the extent to which older people wish to remain near, or move to be near, family members on whom they rely (Finch, 1989). Greece, in contrast, is divided between those older people who have followed younger relatives to the conurbations and those who have remained in or returned to rural areas; on some islands (for example, in the eastern Aegean) the proportion of people aged over 65 years is 30 per cent (Triantafillou and Mestheneos, 1990, p. 11). So there is a range of what constitutes 'typicality' in terms of the geographical location of older people in the family in these two countries.

Second, there is the question of what older people 'do' within the family. It has been noted that in the nuclear family their position should be regarded in terms of relationship rather than role *vis à vis* other family members. Even taking this distinction into account, however, it is important to recognise the diverse ways in which older people both give to and receive from their kin. Research, especially in the UK, has tended to focus on elderly people as dependents within the family (Finch, 1989; Parker, 1990). Yet older members of families, possibly at different stages in the life-cycle, are providers of child-care, of advice and support, and of financial help in families (Finch, 1989; Triantafillou and Mestheneos, 1990). The stress on elderly family members as dependents, in the UK more than in Greece, seems to arise from a combination of a rapid rise in the numbers of 'older elderly' people (aged over 75 years, who are more likely to need care) with a fall in the numbers of younger people (a phenomenon discussed in Chapter 1). In Greece there is a greater emphasis on the contribution made by elderly people to the family, emphasised by tradition, although this appears to be modifying as the population profile ages (Triantafillou and Mestheneos, 1990; Sant Cassia, 1992).

Third, there appears to be a greater similarity in the gender divisions within families in these two countries. In both, men are more likely than women to be regarded as needing some degree of care from other family members, and are likely to receive it at a lower level of dependence (Groves and Finch, 1985; Hicks, 1988; Teperoglou *et al.*, 1990). In both countries, also, this occurs in the context of greater longevity for women than for men, so that the very old are more likely to be women (Zarras, 1980; Finch and Groves, 1982; Jefferys and Thane, 1989; Teperoglou *et al.*, 1990). The work performed by women and men in caring is also likely to be distinct, with men less involved in direct personal caring (such as laundry and bathing) and more involved with indirect tasks (such as house maintenance and financial affairs) (Evandrou, 1990; Triantafillou *et al.*, 1986). So the contemporary family cannot be said to be an equal experience for older men and older women in either country.

Fourth, the future pattern of family relationships in the UK seems less easy to predict, because of the increase in divorce in recent years. Although many who divorce later marry again (indeed, *because* of this fact), it appears probable that patterns of family relationships will become increasingly complex (Finch, 1989; Lewis *et al.*, 1991). What is not clear is how this will affect cross-generational relationships, especially between grandparents and grandchildren, although there is some evidence that divorce does not necessarily terminate such links, or even those between in-laws (Finch, 1989). Because of the influence of the Orthodox Church in Greece, divorce is much less common than in the UK, especially in rural areas, and without further evidence it is not possible to say whether or not such a change would have similar effects (Triantafillou *et al.*, 1986; Stathopoulos and Amera, 1992).

In summary, the 'nuclear family with extensions' may be said to be the predominant set of social relationships in both countries within which elderly people are located. It is an important focus for older people both to give and receive support and help. In both countries there are gender divisions which affect who does and who receives what in the family, with forms of patriarchy evident in both contexts. The impact of divorce is more pronounced in the UK, making it less clear than in Greece how the family relationships of older people will be structured in the near future.

Political economy

Taken as a whole, Europe is an industrialised part of the world. However, within Europe there are major distinctions, and within this dimension Greece and the UK differ considerably. Both the scale and the range of industry and commerce are much greater in the UK than in Greece. Even agriculture in the former may be said to be industrialised in comparison with the partially capitalist and partially peasant agriculture in the latter. As we have seen above, a major impact of industrialisation on the definition of ageing has been the idea of retirement and the associated provision of pensions.

A state-sponsored pension scheme has existed in the UK since the first decade of the twentieth century, and it has subsequently been bolstered for some older people by employment based schemes which in many respects (for example, the age payable) are modelled on the state programme (Phillipson, 1982; Walker, 1986a). The Greek pension system is somewhat different, in that many occupations have developed their own social insurance programmes which include retirement pensions. There are 325 such organisations (*tameia syntaxiouchon*) of which four serve over 96 per cent of the population (Dontas *et al.*, 1991). These organisations provide health insurance as well as pensions, services which are separated in the UK. For those not otherwise covered there is a residual scheme of the Social Insurance Institute (Zarras, 1980; Stathopoulos and Amera, 1992). As a result there are wide variations in the pension provisions for retired Greek workers, including the age of retirement.

The location and type of industry also has a bearing on the experience of older people. In urban industrial areas there are more likely to be supporting public services and, as we have seen, families. Public services are more dispersed in rural areas, even where innovative schemes have been specifically developed (see, for example, Macleod and Smith, 1982). At the same time, rural areas are likely to have higher proportions of older people by whom such services may be required. This applies in the UK outside the metropolitan areas, as well as to much of Greece outside greater Athens and Thessaloniki. In such areas older people may not be isolated from immediate kin or community, but their access to wider kin and public services may be curtailed compared with urban elderly people (Wenger, 1984).

A common factor among these areas is their importance in post-industrial economic developments. In addition to agriculture, the major economic activity of Greece and the non-metropolitan parts of the UK may be said to be tourism (Pantelouris, 1987; Urry, 1990). The level of tourism in Greece is such that the annual number of foreign visitors is now close to 50 per cent of the total indigenous population, and in rural areas of the UK a similar phenomenon has emerged, with the influx of tourists adding massively to local populations.

The major effect tourism may have on local life relating to the circumstances and needs of older people is that it is seasonal. This factor carries implications for the demand placed on local infrastructure (including public services such as medicine), or even for the supply of services which may be introduced specifically for the tourist trade. Those who gain the main economic benefit from tourism (whether workers or owners of services) may well not be resident all year, or may have relocated into the area in order to work in tourism. So the impact of tourism for resident older people may be in disruption rather than the benefit of increased economic activity.

It is important, therefore, to recognise the implications of economic structural divisions within any country, because of the possibility that they will affect older people differently from younger people. The circumstances of elderly people in rural areas are influenced not by the absence of industry, but by the presence of tourism .

The modern democratic state has come to respond to elderly people as 'ex-workers', compared to other possible social constructions, particularly in the provision of income maintenance through pensions. However, the exact forms these and other welfare services have taken in the two countries reflect not only their recent histories, but also the present political structures and the economic problems that have been faced in recent decades. Both countries have experienced what has come to be known as 'fiscal crisis' (O'Connor, 1973), associated with a breakdown (in the UK) or non-emergence after earlier indications of a start (in Greece) of confidence and consensus in the legitimacy of state involvement in public welfare (Mishra, 1984; Petmesidou and Tsoulouvis, 1991). Because their backgrounds are not the same, the outcomes in the two countries are different. In the UK, with a post-war tradition of an extensive welfare state, this crisis has been experienced through a reshaping of welfare provided through the 1980s. A particular feature of these changes has been an attempt to reduce state involvement, through support for increased private provision in health, in social care and in pensions. Greece, in contrast, began to develop a fuller welfare state in the 1980s, including non-contributory pensions for elderly people in rural areas, and some state hospitals and health services including specific services for older people (Pantelouris, 1987; Teperoglou *et al.*, 1990; Dontas *et al.*, 1991). However, such growth was limited and towards the end of the 1980s and in the early years of the 1990s it slowed considerably. The Greek welfare state remains only partially developed, or may even be said to have failed to make more than a minimal beginning (Dontas *et al.*, 1991; Petmesidou and Tsoulouvis, 1991).

In both countries, the failure of welfare state legitimacy is associated with the rise of the New Right in the New Democracy (*Nea Dheemokratia*) and the Conservative parties. The ideological roots of this broad political spectrum (which is evident across Europe and North America) are classical liberalism and include an antipathy to state involvement in civil society. This strengthens a residual view of the welfare state, in which there is no unitary status of older people in need. Rather we can see the emergence of discrimination between those who may be regarded as 'deserving' and those who may not, just as with younger people in comparable circumstances.

In summary, the economic and political structures of Greece and the UK appear to be converging to some degree. Although the extent of industrialisation in either the manufacturing or tourism sectors remains distinct for the two countries as a whole, there appears to be growing similarity of impact on elderly people in urban and rural areas. Also, the political changes associated with the New Right seem to have created the beginnings of divergence in the extent and forms of state welfare. I want to turn now to a brief comparison of the types of contemporary welfare provision in the two countries.

Health and welfare

As I have already begun to indicate, the patterns of pensions and other welfare services provision differs between Greece and the UK in several respects. Broadly, the main distinction is one of coverage and uniformity, related to the length of development and the structural background. Welfare outside the family in Greece is defined by piecemeal arrangements located mostly outside state institutions, in non-governmental organisations, although supported by the state through various direct and indirect financial arrangements (Dontas, 1987; Dontas *et al.*, 1991). In the UK the majority of formal provision is through state institutions, nationally and locally, including pensions, health services, personal social services and, to a lesser extent, specialist housing (Bytheway, 1980). The widespread but small-scale voluntary (that is, non-governmental) organisations are usually regarded as a supplement or alternative to the state provision.

The Greek government has recognised officially the importance of older people as an issue in the implementation of social policy, through the creation of a separate Division for the Protection of the Aged in the Ministry of Health, Welfare and Social Security (Dontas *et al.*, 1991). The equivalent ministries in the UK, namely the Department of Health, and the Scottish, Welsh and Northern Ireland Offices do not have such a focus; the work of the Department of Social Security which is age-related is concerned solely with retirement pensions. Such divisions are replicated at the local level. In the UK the governmental involvement in the welfare of elderly people is divided institutionally along professional and organisational lines (for example, in the division between health and personal social services) rather than focusing on older people themselves. (The Departments of Education and Science (DES) and the Environment (DOE) may be added to this list). It is possible to argue that any distinction of older people at policy level is discriminatory, and that each area should recognise their needs, as with any other 'subgroup' (Bornat *et al.*, 1985). However, the greater concentration in Greek public administration on the needs of older people has enhanced the level of attention given to them in social policy, even though this has been severely limited by wider political factors, as are discussed above. Moreover, as in the UK, several ministries still have operational responsibility for policy areas which affect older people.

From the earlier workhouses, much of the formal state provision in the UK has grown and divided into geriatric facilities within the National Health Service and personal social services such as residential care, day centres and domiciliary care, along with sheltered housing schemes (By the-way, 1980; Fennell *et al.*, 1988). Greece also has seen the development of specialist services, but these are concentrated in the areas of health and income maintenance, with sparse provision of personal social services in comparison to many other European countries (Dontas *et al.*, 1991; Henrard, 1991). In practice, much health provision is also provided in services designed for the general adult population, and this, rather than being explicitly anti-ageist, may at times reflect a lack of attention to or sympathy for the needs of elderly people (Triantafillou and Mestheneos, 1990).

In both countries the roles of professionals have been central to the growth of formal services. These professions also are more developed in the UK than in Greece, with a well-demarcated medical speciality of geriatrics, and other professions such as social work more firmly established in this area (Henrard, 1991), although these professional groups may have low or even marginal status when compared with those concerned with younger adults (for example see Brearley, 1978, and Brocklehurst, 1978). As both countries can be said to have a professionally centred view of health and welfare, the extent and the type of services available are limited because of the relative status of these professional specialisations (Brearley, 1978; Biggs, 1989; Dontas *et al.*, 1991).

Recent trends in both countries, related to the impact of the crisis of welfare legitimacy and the influence of the 'new right' are for an increased emphasis on informal welfare provision (Warnes, 1987a; Finch, 1989; Amira, 1990; Dontas *et al.*, 1991). This takes the form of ideological encouragements for 'the family' to be seen as the primary source and location of care, and for non-family care to be provided either through voluntary organisations or (where possible) through private arrangements rather than directly by the state. Yet the state retains a role, more strongly in the UK, in the support of non-governmental services. This is achieved through subsidies (either as grants to individuals or as tax advantages in making contributions), in the regulation of standards of service, with associated licensing or registration, and in the form of other policy initiatives (including income maintenance benefits) to encourage or compel family members to undertake caring work.

The emphasis within professional services is also changing, from a past concentration on institutional forms of provision towards 'care in the community'. In the UK this has been criticised as a device either to enable privatisation to take place or to place the burden of care on to the families of elderly people, especially women members, by removing alternative sources of support (Finch and Groves, 1980; Ungerson, 1987; Hicks, 1988), and there are implications that a similar perspective could be applied to Greece (Teperoglou *et al.*, 1990; Triantafillou and Mestheneos, 1990).

So, in summary, these two countries, starting from different bases, appear to be converging to a degree in relation to health and welfare policy, around the themes of 'domestic care' and 'privatisation'. The dominance of professionals evident in both countries seems unlikely to be reduced by these developments; rather they provide an alternative context in which professional and non-professional skills and interests in assistance to older people are mixed in the patterns of services available. Reflecting their relationship with the state, professionals exercise considerable influence in the definition of health and welfare (Hugman, 1991), and this is replicated in both Greece and the UK. The connection between these similarities and the membership by both of the European Community is an issue which will be explored further when making comparisons with other countries in later chapters.

A Model Framework

Outline framework

In this chapter, through a comparison of two European countries, I have begun to develop the themes which will constitute the basis for a comparative framework. In this final section I will draw out specific points to define the framework, which will be developed successively in the following chapters.

The first element I have identified is that of *history and culture*. In this discussion it was seen that although there are some similarities in the historical dimensions of old age (even to the point that one culture explicitly makes reference to aspects of the history of the other), nevertheless there are important differences. The implications of industrialisation, colonialism and other political factors, religion and the family combine in contemporary social circumstances to make the reality of old age different in Greece and the UK. But how do these differ across Europe? What impact have they had on the variety of experience of and responses to old age in European society? These questions will be explored out in the first part of the wider comparison.

international study of ageing. Yet they do so in encyclopaedic form, visiting each country in turn, in the manner of a 'tourist guide' (Kraan *et al.*, 1991, p. 6). Little (1979, pp. 149–53) is an exception, developing a comparative method based on the conceptual distinction between 'residual' and 'institutional' forms of social response to dependency needs in old age. This is used to produce a continuum of types of welfare for older people, on which countries are placed according to the extent and type of provision available from the most 'residual' (Afghanistan) to the most 'institutional' (Sweden). As Little herself notes (1979, p. 149), the advantages of being able to categorise countries on the same basis has to be set against the limitations of not being able to take into account the subtleties of urbanisation, recent history and so on. So I do not want to follow Little's model, as these are important criteria which will be developed later in this chapter. Similarly, the distinction made by Kosberg (1992) between countries as 'young, youthful, adult, mature and aged' in relation to the proportions of older people in their populations is limited on these grounds, although it forms the basis for a challenge to the modernisation thesis. This is not to deny that the frameworks of Little and of Kosberg do provide useful comparative data, on which I will draw in subsequent chapters.

More recently, several studies have developed distinctions of societies in terms of welfare state responses to older people. Titmuss's (1963) categorisation of welfare states as 'residual', 'industrial achievement–performance' and 'institutional–redistributive' has informed work in France, Germany, Scandinavia and the UK (Jamieson, 1990; Evers and Olk, 1991). These categories approximate to conservative, liberal and socialist models of welfare states and as such relate to wider debates (Esping-Andersen, 1990). Yet Evers and Olk (1991, pp. 77–8) identify the main weakness of this approach, which is one shared to an extent by all conceptual frameworks, that no country can be fitted easily into a single category. The usual assignation of Germany, the UK and Denmark to each category respectively is limited, they argue, because all these countries now have mixed systems. However, the strength of this approach is in the detail with which a small number of examples can be explored in relation to a common theme. (I will return to the 'welfare mix' in Chapter 7.)

All these studies of old age and older people can be placed within the continuum of comparative approaches outlined by Jones (1985), from a series of discrete case studies through to a generalised discussion using illustrative examples. The place any study occupies on this continuum is based on its purposes, from detailed empirical enquiries into specific areas of policy and practice through to general theory-building approaches looking at wider issues. Jones, in common with Shanas *et al.* (1968), argues that

Second, images of ageing and the social value ascribed to old age are ambivalent, historically and in the present, in both countries. This raises the question of the extent to which older people can be said to be *respected or abused* in the different national societies of Europe. Concern with the actual 'abuse' of elderly people, especially by carers, whether formal or informal, is a part of this issue. It has become a matter of public and academic debate in North America and more recently in the UK (Eastman, 1984). The concern about 'abuse' of older people (which includes, but is not confined to physical violence) is closely interwoven with wider social attitudes to old age. In the second part of the wider discussion, therefore, I will examine the evidence for the occcurence of this phenomenon across Europe, and look at its relationship with more general images of ageing.

The third aspect of the comparative framework has been identified in the preceding discussion of the *welfare responses to elderly people*. It has been noted that these differ with respect to the social and political context in which they are located, but that in both countries they are dominated by the interests of professionals. To what extent is this pattern to be seen across Europe? Who organises and who uses welfare services? Do these services in turn create old age either as a concept or as an experience for people? These questions will be explored in the third part of the broader comparison.

In the fourth part of the framework I want to turn to a quite specific issue which has been identified in the comparison of Greece and the UK, and which, it has been suggested, has wider significance. This is the relationship between *institutions and communities* in the provision of health and welfare services to older people. Some similarities between Greece and the UK have been discussed in this chapter, and it will be necessary to further ask whether this is a social division which has meaning across Europe or whether it is a construction which applies only to some countries. The variety of patterns emerging in different parts of Europe is also an important factor.

The utility of the framework

Although it is my purpose, as I argued above, to develop a comparative understanding of ageing and the welfare of older people, I do not intend to confine myself to anthropological, historical or sociological enquiries. While I agree that any concern with old age should be informed by such approaches, ageing and older people are firmly on the political and profes-sional agenda and it is my aim also to address these questions. Therefore the discussion will additionally be directed to issues of policy and profes-sional action, subjecting these to the same degree of analysis as that applied to the situation of the older people they have been developed to serve. In the final chapter, examples of specific policies and service developments will be used to illustrate the wider issues.

I think, also, that the comparative method of enquiry has an applied dimension. One approach to learning is to contrast a range of possibilities, and in a field where there is a considerable prejudging of knowledge and issues, a mutual exchange of ideas and practices may help in the elaboration of new responses to the situation of older people in our societies. If nothing else, it may remind us that no one has thought of everything: professionals, policy-makers and researchers in different European countries have much to learn from each other as well as from older people themselves. In the concluding chapter I will examine the degree of convergence and the possibilities for mutual learning about ageing and the welfare of older people in Europe.

3

History, Economy and Culture

Socio-Political Aspects of the Construction of Ageing

Relativity: time and space

In the comparison of Greece and the UK in the previous chapter issues of industrialisation urbanisation and the associated complexities of social order and relationship were identified as important factors for understanding the background to and experience of the lives of older people. What it means to be old was seen as relative to the period and the geographical location of the older person. I want now to explore the widen implications across Europe of these factors for ageing. I will look first at sociopolitical issues, of which industrialisation (and consequent urbanisation) has been identified by many gerontologists as a crucial explanatory dimension in the history of ageing (Scott Smith, 1982; Guillemard, 1983; Fennell *et al.*, 1988). Questions of colonialism, migration and war will also be addressed. This brings our discussion back to the debate between modernisation, demography and political economy as explanations of change (Scott Smith, 1982). Following from this I will examine more widely other aspects of social development, including religion and other cultural factors, and the family – which, although in a sense 'cultural', represents a distinct and important area of social structures, organisation and relationships warranting separate analysis. This discussion will form the basis for the examination of policy and professional responses in the following chapters.

Economy and industrialisation

The phenomenon of increasing proportions of older people in urban industrial societies of Europe compared with the rural preindustrial world has been widely documented over a long period (Stearns, 1977, pp. 15–16,

42; Minois, 1989, pp. 289–90). This demographic development may be attributed largely to the increase in life expectancy arising from improved health and hygiene, especially in childbirth; and there have been more people surviving the particularly dangerous period of infancy and child-hood, along with a particularly marked increase in life expectancy for women (Minois, 1989, pp. 291–3). While these demographic changes cannot be attributed solely to industrialisation, they can be associated with the nascent development of science and technology which subsequently gave rise to the Industrial Revolution in north-western Europe.

Industrialisation did not have a uniform effect on what has come to be regarded as the ageing of the population (for example, see Victor, 1987, p. 103). Indeed, during the main periods of industrialisation in England, France, Germany and The Netherlands, the proportion of older people (defined as aged over 60 years) declined slightly (Stearns, 1977; Minois, 1989). However, this may be accounted for by the moderately increased life expectancy of younger people in that period and, perhaps more, by the level of fertility rates compared to mortality rates, which remained high until the end of the nineteenth century (Victor, 1987).

It was in the late nineteenth century and into the twentieth that the demographic trends turned sharply, and the proportions of people aged over 65 years in the industrialised countries that are now part of the EC reached their current relatively high proportions of between approximately 11 and 16 per cent (Eurostat, 1991). This has generated the explanation that it is *post*-industrialism rather than industrialism that has brought benefits of markedly increased life expectancy. The 1990 figures shown in Table 3.1 indicate that Belgium, Denmark, Germany and the UK (countries which had early industrialisation) are at the higher end of the range, compared with Portugal, Spain and Eire at the other. France, Italy and Greece lie in the middle, but for very different reasons. France and Italy are countries which have partially industrialised and partly retained a more rural, agri-cultural base (both countries having a rough North–South divide in this respect). Greece, though later to industrialise and urbanise, like Portugal or Spain, has been affected greatly by emigration during the twentieth century in comparison to the other countries of the 'Mediterranean rim'. The coun-try which does not otherwise fit this pattern is The Netherlands – uncharac-teristically for an industrialised nation, this has a 'youthful' population (Pijl, 1992).

The other Scandinavian countries industrialised at a comparatively late date but rapidly became affluent. Their relative populations aged over 65 years are: Finland, 12.9 per cent (1987); Norway, 16.3 per cent (1990); and Sweden, 18.3 per cent (1988) (United Nations, 1992).

TABLE 3.1 *Proportions of total populations aged over 65 years, EC countries, 1990*

Country	Percentage over 65	Relative order
Belgium	14.8	4
Denmark	15.6	1=
France	14.0	6
Germany	15.3	3
Greece	13.7	7
Irish Republic	11.3	12
Italy	14.5	5
Luxembourg	13.4	8
The Netherlands	12.8	11
Portugal	13.1	10
Spain	13.3	9
United Kingdom	15.6	1=

Source: Eurostat, 1991.

In the more agricultural countries of Eastern Europe and the Mediterranean, with later industrialisation, similar patterns also appear to be emerging. Indicative percentage populations over 65 years are: Bulgaria, 12.8 (1989); Cyprus, 10.2 (1989); Czechoslovakia 11.7 (1989); Hungary 13.2 (1989); Malta 10.3 (1989); and Poland 9.7 (1988) (United Nations, 1992). In comparison, Turkey (also a Council of Europe member and seeking entry to the EC) is considerably less industrialised and demonstrates a demographic profile closer to countries such as India or Iraq, with 4.2 per cent of its population aged over 65 years in 1985 (Gilleard *et al.*, 1985; United Nations, 1992).

Industrialisation is therefore associated in Europe with both the rise in longevity and the ageing profile of populations, but in respect of the changes it brings in its wake, rather than as part of the process. There are three reasons why this may be so. The first is that the material benefits of industrial society enhance longer life expectancy, with increased health and wealth as industrial society becomes established: food becomes more plentiful and varied, the water cleaner and in more guaranteed supply, working hours are reduced, and housing becomes generally better, as does medical care, which is also more widely available. The second reason is that the ageing of society is a proportional change, and this arises from lower fertility at the same time as increased longevity. There is no longer a necessity (whether this is defined economically or culturally) for large numbers of children per family, because the expectation that all will survive to adulthood is so much greater. At the same time, contraceptive technologies make reduced fertility a more widely available option. (The low usage of available contraception in developing countries must be considered a qualifying factor here.) Third, industrialisation has created patterns of consumption in which small family size maximises opportunities. So, the ageing of Europe derives from falling birth-rates and falling death-rates; both are the product of advanced industrialisation.

Industrialisation has affected not only how many older people there are in European society, but also their social roles and status. Through the Industrial Revolution, the social nature of old age has been shaped within the growth of capitalism (Phillipson, 1982). As I noted in Chapter 1, the modernisation thesis argues that, as the factory replaced the field or the home as the centre of paid work, the social status of older people change from that of 'wise elder' or 'the triumphant survivor' to that of 'the ex-worker'. To what extent is this the case? Are older people no longer defined by what they are, prized even if grudgingly, but by what they are not, in a denigrated, surplus role?

Rural and urban life

To begin to answer these questions, the first issue is the status of older people in rural agrarian society. There appears to be a wide historical diversity across Europe in the economic status of older people. Quadagno (1982) considers evidence from the UK and Denmark, noting that the status of older people might frequently be ambiguous in agrarian life. In particular, the control older people in rural society might exercise over their offspring was a tangible source of power, but could lead to resentment and inter-generational conflict if either party did not adhere to agreements, for example by parents holding on to land necessary for a son to marry, or by offspring not taking care of parents who had relinquished land. A similar situation existed in Sweden (Andersson, 1992). This is an example of the pattern discussed in Chapter 2, in which older people exert power through control of material and symbolic resources, and it has been argued that the inter-generational frictions produced by such relationships was a major contributory factor to the association of older people with miserliness (Covey, 1991). Under factory employment in the urban context such rigid inter-generational roles were no longer possible, although for the emerging capitalist class this issue might survive in a different form and inheritance continue to be important. For example, Lowy (1979) noted that in the (pre-unification) Federal Republic of Germany most of the 10 per cent of people aged over 65 years still in the labour force were either agricultural workers or self-employed. Similar employment patterns have also been discerned in France and Denmark in the recent past, while in contemporary Poland the figure remains as high as 97 per cent in some areas (Shanas *et al.*, 1968; Huet and Fontaine, 1980; Hrynkiewicz *et al.*, 1991).

Again, the countries of the north and west of Europe (with the exception of the Irish Republic) may be distinguished from those of the south and east in the relationship between these changes and the status of the majority of older people. The strength of inter-generational links in the south and east appears to be associated with later industrialisation and the slower pace of change in agricultural areas (Lisón-Tolosana, 1976; Sant Cassia, 1992). However, it is important to distinguish in all countries between different regions because, for example, the industrialised towns and cities of Greece or Italy resemble those of Germany or the UK in this respect (Florea, 1980; Dontas, 1987; Bianchi, 1991).

The recognition of regional diversity within countries suggests another dimension to the development of ageing and old age, and that is urbanisation. In the more industrial countries in the 1970s the majority of older people were likely to be city dwellers compared to the prevalence of older people in rural areas of the less industrialised countries (Lowy, 1979; Smolic-Krkovic, 1979). More recent evidence suggests that this position is changing with further industrialisation, exemplified by the position in eastern Europe, where recent years have seen a large increase in the number of elderly city dwellers (Hrynkiewicz *et al.*, 1991).

Although the influence of industry can be seen in a comparison between countries, internal variations may point to an associated factor: that manufacturing industry has tended to result in the growth of urban areas with a high density of population. Several studies have suggested that in such circumstances there is a breakdown in the more traditional forms of support offered to older people, with a consequent sense of isolation and loss of role (Pitsiou, 1986; Jylhä and Jokela, 1990; Teperoglou *et al.*, 1990; Castle-Kanerova, 1992; Széman, 1992).

There are two possible reasons for this phenomenon. First, the migration of younger people from rural areas leaves older people more cut off from the younger members of their families. This results in rural areas where, because the proportion of older people rises rapidly, it is not possible to sustain the more traditional forms of family relationship. Isolation is experienced relative to the location of the family members from whom the older person would expect to seek support. This sense of being 'distant from family' is then amplified and maintained by contact with a peer group with which the same ideas are shared. Second, when older people do follow younger family to urban areas, the pace of life, more distant social relationships and other features of the city serve to isolate the older person, who is also cut off from their peer group (Florea, 1980; Zarras, 1980; Pitsiou, 1986; Amira, 1990; Jylhä and Jokela, 1990; Teperoglou *et al.*, 1990; Bianchi, 1991).

However, other studies have argued that if treated too simplistically, this approach can lead to the 'myth of a golden age' for older people in rural society. Considerable evidence has been offered over a long period of time that the majority of older people in urban industrial areas do have frequent contact with kin (Rosenmayr and Köckeis, 1963; Shanas *et al.*, 1968; Victor, 1987; Finch, 1989; Kraan *et al.*, 1991). At the same time, historical studies (as we have seen above) suggest that old age in a rural environment may have been, and may still be, extremely variable in its quality.

Yet the work of Shanas *et al.* (1968, p. 258 ff.) did point to some links between the objective evidence and the subjective experience which would seem to be widespread (and durable, we might note). They showed that large proportions of older people in three advanced industrial countries (Denmark, the UK and the USA) had regular and frequent contact with family and friends. Yet this was interpreted by older people as less than they might reasonably expect in comparison to the lives of younger relatives, with their own lives when slightly younger and with their images of earlier generations (which may or may not have contained an inaccurate 'golden glow'). In each case the comparator appeared to be an idealised model of greater social activity and status, with more widespread networks. Gender was also a factor, with women reporting slightly more isolation than men, as did people who had not married or those who were widowed and did not have children. Victor (1987) identifies a further dimension, in that comparisons with the recollections of earlier generations will be affected by diminishing family size, as the supply of relatives with whom one may interact is changed along with the lifestyles in which they are involved. In short, the comparators are not necessarily similar. I will return to these issues below, in a discussion of the family.

That the strongest contemporary evidence for the modernisation explanation of ageing comes from south and east Europe (Greece, Hungary, Italy, Poland, Portugal, Spain, and so on), where industrialisation and urbanisation are more recent phenomena, lends some credence to the explanation that modernisation constructs ageing as a subjective experience. This is not to deny the problematic nature of old age in rural agrarian life or its idolisation by current generations of older people. What it does suggest is that the rapid urbanisation in these countries in the twentieth century is associated for the current older generation with a different experience of being old than the one they remember anticipating. Thus is it the pace of change, as experienced by the present cohort of older people, which creates the conditions for the feeling that 'old age is not what it used to be' (Cowgill and Holmes, 1972, p. 312).

A particular group of older people for whom ageing in industrial European society may also hold a different reality from that anticipated are elderly members of ethnic minority communities, especially those who have migrated from other parts of the world. In the UK, for instance, the lives of older New Commonwealth and Pakistan immigrants is more likely to be characterised by poverty and isolation than that of older members of the white indigenous communities (Bhalla and Blakemore, 1981; Blakemore, 1985; Norman, 1985). This results partly from patterns of migration (with single men having been the most likely to migrate) as well as from racism and disadvantage in employment and services. In other words, in part the experience of older people in the ethnic minorities in urban European society replicates features of the ethnic majority (being affected by the presence or absence of a spouse and children), while in part it is specific to ethnic minority status (affected by racism). This situation can be seen in other post-colonial countries, such as France, Germany and The Netherlands, although until recently much European research on ageing has tended to ignore issues of ethnicity and racism (Featherstone and Hepworth, 1990; Pijl, 1991). Two associated myths, the 'myth of return' and the 'myth of extensive family care', both play into the discrimination experienced by ethnic minority older people who are settlers and who, despite continuing strong cultures of family obligation in many instances, are less likely than the white majority to have an extensive family network available (Saifullah Khan, 1977; Blakemore, 1985).

Pensions: older people as ex-workers

The second aspect of the debate between modernisation and political economy as explanations of the construction of old age revolves around the introduction of retirement pensions and the creation of the ex-worker as a social role.

In Europe the development of retirement pensions has followed an uneven historical course, with civil servants often having been the first to receive them (in Belgium and The Netherlands in 1844, Germany in 1893), followed by industrial workers (de Beauvoir, 1977). As I noted in Chapter 2, in the UK, pension schemes only related to specific occupations until 1948, while in France well into the twentieth century, pension arrangements were piecemeal (Stearns, 1977; Guillemard, 1983). However, there is now extensive provision in EC member countries, with the state providing basic guaranteed minimum levels of income even where other arrangements are not made (Drury, 1992). For example, retirement pensions were the major source of income for 78 per cent of elderly people in the Federal Republic of Germany, with all older people eligible; in France all retired workers are eligible for income maintenance assistance if their income is below a certain level; in Italy as many as 80 per cent of older people draw the basic 'social pension'; and in Greece there is a residual scheme for those not otherwise covered by the complex network of pension syndicates (Guillemard, 1983; von Ballusek, 1983; Bianchi, 1991; Dontas *et al.*, 1991; Robolis, 1993).

Scandinavian countries also have extensive retirement pension arrangements, and were early providers of state schemes (Havighurst, 1978; Daatland, 1992). These have been extended in recent decades, for example in Denmark where state pension arrangements were expanded in 1956 to cover all people aged over 65, regardless of past or immediate income (Siim, 1990). Outside the EC, Norway and Sweden have flat-rate non-contributory pension systems which ensure a basic standard income for all people over the age of 67 (Wærness, 1990). Daatland (1992) notes that in Norway 71 per cent of the income of pensioners comes from the National Pensions Scheme, and that in all Scandinavian countries pensions are universal and relatively generous.

In Eastern Europe, however, the provision of pensions is less certain. Some older people in the former Yugoslavia, in the recent past, for example, may not have been eligible and so were entirely dependent financially on their families (Smolic-Krkovic, 1979), while some regions still had not implemented compulsory pension schemes by the time of the division of the country and subsequent civil war (Rusica *et al.*, 1991). In Poland in the late 1970s there were also a small number of people, mainly independent farmers, who were not eligible (Synak, 1987a). The situation had not improved by 1990, with rural older people subject to arbitrary entitlements and an average of 25 per cent lower pension levels than former industrial workers (Hrynkiewicz *et al.*, 1991). In this comparison it is difficult to distinguish whether the social policies of communist countries were structured against sections of society, such as independent farmers, or whether their economies were unable to sustain universal minimum pensions in comparison with the capitalist countries. The comments of de Beauvoir (1977) concerning the lack of pensions for retired 'liberal professionals' in Hungary, which is still evident, supports the former interpretation (Széman, 1992). However, the example of Turkey as another country which has defined itself as a potential member of the EC underlines the complexity of generalisation. As in Eastern Europe, the employment of older people is more extensive in rural agricultural than urban industrial areas. At the same time, pensions are available only to about 30 per cent of the workforce as a whole, with a means-tested income maintenance system for people not entitled to a pension; take-up is haphazard (Gurkan and Gilleard 1987).

Retirement is another aspect of ageing in which gender may be seen to be an important dimension, affecting both the age of retirement and the pension arrangements available to the older person (Arber and Ginn, 1991). In some European countries women retire earlier than men, supported by pension entitlements, while in others there is no gender difference in the age at which pensions may be obtained. Table 3.2 shows that in Greece, Italy, Portugal, Spain and the UK, gender discrimination in pensions continue to operate (although the EC is considering a directive on standardisation). Outside the EC, Austria and Switzerland also discriminate, while the Scandinavian countries have parity between women and men (although these countries have different retirement ages from each other) (Drury, 1992). Public policy is a major determinant in this respect, with the provision of state pensions affecting the differential ages of women and men on retirement. However, it is not the only factor, as Havighurst (1978) recorded that in *all* of a selection of European countries (including Scandinavia) as well as North America and Australasia, women were less likely than men to remain in the labour force over the age of 65 years and that this has been the situation for much of the twentieth century: cultural sexism, ageing and work are interconnected (Arber and Ginn, 1991).

TABLE 3.2   *The age at which women and men may obtain retirement pensions, EC countries, 1990*

Country	Women	Men
Belgium	60–65	60–65
Denmark	67	67
France	60	60
Germany	65	65
Greece	60	65
Irish Republic	65	65
Italy	55	60
Luxembourg	65	65
The Netherlands	65	65
Portugal	62	65
Spain	60	65
United Kingdom	60	65

Source: Drury, 1992.

Whether or not women do retire earlier than men, and irrespective of the support given to this phenomenon by pension arrangements, women tend to be disadvantaged in retirement (Groves, 1987; Daatland, 1992). In the UK, for example, married women are still in some respects assumed to be dependent on their husband in pension provision, a situation which previously was buttressed by the possibility for married women of paying a reduced contribution towards state benefits because their economic activity was regarded as secondary. The UK position appears to have been paralleled by the earlier French formation of pensions in male-dominated or exclusive industries, with pressure for contributory schemes so that entitlement could be looked upon as property and so passed to widows and other dependents (Stearns, 1977). Additional pensions for men based on employment is still payable in The Netherlands (Kraan *et al.*, 1991). This situation is a continuation of the marginal position of women in low-paid or part-time work in most European countries, although there have been policy initiatives to equalise benefits (Sanidad y Seguridad, 1981; von Ballusek, 1983; Groves, 1987; Fennell *et al.*, 1988; Leira, 1990; Siim, 1990). The notable exceptions appear to be Sweden, where at the age of 67 some women may be better off than their male counterparts, and Greece where some women may be eligible for additional pension from the age of 55 because of family size (Sheppard and Mullins, 1989; Dontas *et al.*, 1991). The latter example appears to be tied to notions of 'motherhood' and a policy to encourage population growth; it should therefore also be seen as being discriminatory.

The main factor which led originally to the development of retirement pensions can be regarded as the balance of interests between workers and employers (de Beauvoir, 1977; Stearns, 1977; Phillipson, 1982). By this is meant that the 'need' of commerce, administration and industry for younger workers, because of perceived health and adaptability, is balanced by the supposed benefits of not having to endure work for which one may not have a great liking. Yet does this assumption of the eagerness to leave work really hold true? Do people only remain at work out of financial desperation? Where poverty is a likely consequence this may be a powerful reason, but Phillipson (1982), reviewing studies undertaken in the UK, France and The Netherlands, draws attention to the benefits of work (friendship, activity, interest) compared to the benefits of retirement (leisure, independence). Staying at work may be a means of maintaining social contact and one's sense of self where this has been moulded over as many as fifty years in an occupation. Even when retirement *is* regarded as being positive, people who have been in employment for most of their adult life, usually men, may still refer to themselves as 'a retired ...'. Capitalism may be said to create us in the image of our productivity.

Where retirement is a positive experience, it appears that class factors play a considerable part, with office and professional workers more able to continue using work skills in a non-work setting, or having the opportunity to develop other interests, than are manual workers. People in middle-class occupational groups seem to be more able to maintain their sense of self derived from a work identity, and many were observed in a study in the UK to have reduced their amount of passive leisure time (television watching, reading and so on) (Abrams, 1978). A similar observation is made by Wærness (1990) about the relatively easy and positive transition into retirement for both men and women which is demonstrated in Scandinavian research. Evidence from Germany also supports the idea of active retirement, with older people seeking interesting or socially useful ways to spend their time and to make a contribution to society, either through cultural or sporting activities or through the provision of mutual assistance (meals, visiting and so on) (Dieck, 1990).

However, Phillipson (1982, p. 51) notes that such a construction of old age still includes the underlying implication of older people as redundant, in that it is less often about personal development or productivity than about consumption. More recent developments, such as the University of the Third Age (in Belgium, France, Italy, The Netherlands, Portugal and the UK), are a response to this, confronting the idea of old age as a removal from the active part of society (Huet and Fontaine, 1980; Fogarty, 1986; Leeson *et al.*, 1993). Nevertheless, whether positive or negative in its implications for the individual, retirement may construct older people as ex-workers.

Several studies have drawn attention also to the gendered nature of the experience of retirement, noting that it may be different for women and men (de Beauvoir, 1977; Phillipson, 1982; Groves, 1987; Gilbert *et al.*, 1990; Wærness, 1990; Arber and Ginn, 1991). These differences reflect the wider social discrimination between women and men in employment, family roles and public services. For some women retirement may never take place, as domestic work is ever-present; others may experience retirement vicariously through their partner; and for yet other women, a reluctance to retire from paid employment may be experienced as strongly as that evident among some men, and for the same reasons. Moreover, although there appear to be few gender differences in whether partners provide care for each other in older age (the types of care may differ), when other members of the family are concerned women are more likely than men to be involved in the unpaid work of caring for someone else, soon after retirement or even giving up work in order to be a carer (Hicks, 1988; Finch, 1989; Evandrou, 1990; Evers and Olk, 1991). The availability of professional care services has an impact on this, and the presence of such services accounts for differences in experience between women in the various countries of Europe, such as the greater availability of services in Scandinavia compared with the UK, and either of these compared with countries of the 'Mediterranean rim' (Hicks, 1988; Leira, 1990; Teperoglou *et al.*, 1990).

Colonialism and migration

A major political influence on the social construction of ageing in Europe has been the rise and fall of colonialism, in which some countries have been colonisers while others have been colonised. These different histories create diverse backgrounds for the meaning of old age within various national societies. In previous Chapter 2 I noted that while in the UK (a colonial power) immigration from former colonies has created a multicultural context in which there is a range of interpretations of ageing, which in turn is affected by racism, in Greece (a former colony) the understanding of old age is bound up with national history and independence. Most of the countries of Europe, particularly in the north and west, are former colonial powers; those EC countries which have been colonised in the last two centuries are the Irish Republic and Greece.

A crucial distinction between colonising and colonised countries has been in terms of cross-national migration and its impact on demographic structures. Both the Irish Republic and Greece are characterised by population loss during the twentieth century as younger people emigrated in search of employment, with North America and Australia being the main destinations (Fleetwood, 1980; Dontas et al., 1991). In this sense they appear to parallel the post-colonial countries of Africa, America and Asia in that they have formed a supply of industrial labour for other nations. However, to the extent that the Irish Republic and Greece have also themselves industrialised, the demographic impact of emigration has been different from that in Africa or Asia, creating much more rapidly ageing populations with overall profiles that match the more highly industrialised countries (see page 48). The peculiarity of this history also plays a part in shaping the more rural location of many older people in the Irish Republic and Greece (in the early 1990s) in the areas which younger people have left. The possibility for elderly people of following younger relatives, which exists with internal migration from the west coast to Dublin, or from the islands to Athens, is not such an easy option if the younger relatives are in Chicago or Melbourne.

The former colonial powers, such as France, Germany, Italy and The Netherlands, share the experience of the UK as the receivers of immigrant

labour from former colonies (Zapf, 1986). However, as this has been predominantly in the last forty years, the impact on the elderly population has
been relatively slight. The post-colonial settlers for the most part have been
of working age on arrival, and although they may be growing old in Europe
they do not, as yet, form the same proportion of the community as do older
White Europeans (Norman, 1985; Paillat, 1989; Pijl, 1992). The situation
in Germany has been characterised by the more transient tradition of 'guest
workers' (*gästarbeiter*), with smaller numbers of migrant workers settling
when compared to France, The Netherlands and the UK (Zapf, 1986).
Nevertheless, it is possible to identify issues of racism in the ambivalent
responses of white Europeans to black elderly people. For example,
assumptions about norms of family and other informal care within minority
ethnic communities can lead to simultaneous perceptions of 'being over-
demanding' or 'unreasonably refusing' public services (Bhalla and
Blakemore, 1981; Torkington, 1983; Norman, 1985; Cameron *et al.*, 1989;
Williams, 1990). Concentrations of black older people, for example in
some French and UK cities, may also give a false impression to policy-
makers and professionals (Paillat, 1989). However, the numbers of ethnic
minority elderly people in European society will continue to rise, and challenging the racism inherent in responses to black older people seems likely
to remain a political issue into the twenty-first century (Pijl, 1991).

For a minority of Europeans, therefore, the relationship between ageing
and migration is of some importance. Ageing has shaped the *experience* of
migration, while migration has shaped the *context* of ageing, particularly as
a consequence of colonialism and its aftermath.

More recent migration within Europe is also creating a situation in
which the position of older people may become contentious through its
impact on the economics of ageing. This is highlighted by the positions of
Germany and Greece in relation to an influx of migrant workers from Eastern Europe (Stathopoulos and Amera, 1992; Fischer, 1993). Similarly,
Luxembourg as the administrative centre of the EC, now has approximately 25 per cent of its population foreign-born (Paillat, 1989). In both
instances, the prospect is that the impact on pension provision will be the
factor which makes the link between migration and ageing contentious into
the twenty-first century.

War

The scale of war in Europe increased markedly during the twentieth
century (again as a consequence of industrialisation), not only in the First
World War (the 'Great War') of 1914–18 and the Second World War of

1939–45, but also a series of more minor wars and conflicts fought within Europe and by European states elsewhere in the world. This means that everyone born before 1927 in every European country has been an adult (defined as aged over 18 years) while their country has been involved in at least one major conflict. The implications of this are likely to be seen not only in the subjective experiences and expectations of older people (for example, in the earlier deaths of relatives and friends) but also in the demographic structures of age groups in which relatively large numbers of people were killed. Synak (1987b) argues that some parts of Europe (particularly central European countries such as Poland) are more likely to be affected by this because of the scale of killing which took place between 1939 and 1945. The instance Synak gives is of an unusually high ratio of women to men in Poland in the age cohorts over 65 years compared to other European countries, reflecting gender divisions in military action (Synak, 1987b, p. 23). A similar phenomenon is noted by Amann (1980a) and Hörl (1992) in Austria. The population figures for the Central European countries of Austria, Czechoslovakia, Hungary and Poland all show such an impact in that the cohorts currently aged 70–74 are smaller than those aged 75–79 (United Nations, 1992), contrary to normal expectations, which may also be ascribed to the demographic effects of major war.

Social gerontology has made little reference to the demographic impact of war. As Synak (1987b) recognises, any conclusions have to be based on comparison, either between countries or over time. So this lacuna is understandable because it is only in the late 1990s, as the first European generation of this century not to have been part of major conflict reaches retirement age, that any such implications are likely to be detectable (Grundy and Harrop, 1992). For example, the detailed sex differences of life expectancy may be affected by this factor, although other changes (in particular the move away from a heavy-industry base) may also have an impact. Older people in the countries of the former Yugoslavia may possibly be an exception to this, as at the time of writing genocide is occurring in the struggles for post-Communist independence. In the remainder of Europe, the cohort of those who were young adults during the 1939–45 war will reach the age of 75 years between the years 1996 and 2002, so it will be in the twenty-first century that firmer conclusions may be possible.

Demography and modernity in industrialisation

It appears that, as regards industrialisation and urbanisation, there is a risk of overstating the opposition of demography and modernisation to political economy as explanatory theses. This overview has noted that while the objective increase in both the numbers and the proportions of older people in European countries is a general demographic trend, the subjective experience of ageing is shaped by these demographic factors in relation to issues of modernism. To this extent I would wish to suggest that both concepts are relevant to the understanding of sociopolitical factors as they affect ageing in Europe. Nevertheless, both demographic trends and issues of modernisation are grounded in the social, economic and political relationships which form the context for the lives of older people. The social construction of the ex-worker within the more individualised pattern of urban social relationships provides a central example. It seems appropriate, therefore, to continue to use insights from those perspectives while placing them within an overall structural social theory in which the nature of industrial and post-industrial capitalism are placed centre-stage.

Cultural Aspects in the Construction of Ageing

Religion and ageing

At the core of the modernisation concept as an explanation for experiences of ageing in modern society is the assumption of a loss of status for older people in recent history. This is based in large part on the evidence of changes which had taken place in religious and other cultural constructions of old age and social responses to older people (Cowgill, 1972; Fischer, 1978; Silverman and Maxwell, 1982). To explore further the wider relevance of this assumption I want to look first at religion and then at other aspects of European culture.

In Chapter 2 I noted that some historians and sociologists have made connections between forms of religion, capitalism and modernism. Tawney (1926) and Weber (1930) both identified connections between the development of Protestant Christianity and industrial capitalism through the wider social and cultural changes which took place in northern Europe (Bendix, 1966; Eldridge, 1971). Following these later commentators, I want to be clear that I do not take either Weber or Tawney to be explaining capitalism as a consequence of religious change, but noting that there is an interconnection, in which each is buttressed by and shaped against the development of the other. So, for instance, although nascent capitalism was evident also in Roman Catholic areas, its impact was filtered through a different religious philosophy which bound it more closely to traditional social structures and relationships. These, it may be inferred, included social constructions surrounding old age.

Implications of industrialisation for old age have been examined above. What differences in the social construction of and responses to ageing can be identified between European countries on the basis of their *religious* heritage? Is there a distinction between the Protestant 'north', the Roman Catholic 'south' and the Orthodox 'east' of Europe overlapping the patterns of industrial development?

At face value there may appear to be such a connection, for example in the extent of state involvement in the care of dependent older people which is greatest in countries with a Protestant heritage (associated with individualism and privatisation in the moral order) compared to Roman Catholic or Orthodox countries (associated with communalism in the moral order). In relation to the origins of welfare state policies and the penetration of civil society by the welfare state there appears to be evidence of such a connection. It is in Germany, The Netherlands, the UK and (perhaps most notably) the Scandinavian countries that the earlier forms of welfare state development can be seen (Kraan *et al.*, 1991), and in which the idea of citizenship is widely accepted as the basis of the relationship between the individual and the state (Taylor, 1989). This includes the provision of basic pensions, health care and social welfare services (Hunter, 1986; Midre and Synak, 1989; Henrard, 1991; Daatland, 1992). In contrast, the state has had a very limited role in welfare developments in a country such as Greece, where citizenship in this sense is not understood and where the state is perceived to be an alien construction against which people make demands (Dontas *et al.*, 1991; Petmesidou and Tsoulouvis, 1991).

The connection with religious history, however, is one of association rather than causality. Not only are there Roman Catholic countries (such as France and Italy) where welfare states have developed, albeit in different forms, but other phenomena run counter to a simple causal connection of religious and philosophical thought to social constructions of, and responses to, ageing. The development of pensions could be regarded as an expression of an individualised sense of responsibility for those who no longer work (associated with Protestantism) as compared to the corporate and social models of Roman Catholicism or Orthodoxy. However, as we have already seen, pensions developed at an early stage in France and Belgium as well as in Germany, The Netherlands, the UK and Scandinavia, in response to the political economy of industrialisation rather than the ideological construction of concern for the welfare of older people. For this reason it would appear to be more plausible to regard religious thought as part of the complex of social forces acting to create specific responses to old age, but not one which can be seen as causal.

At the same time it would be incorrect to conclude that the greater secularisation of society arising from the Protestant Reformation necessarily translates into a cessation of church involvement in the care of older people and the moulding of old age. What is more apparent is that such involvement is exercised through the mechanism of voluntary organisations which exist (perhaps even compete) on comparable terms with organisations that do not have a religious basis. This is an expression of modernism as described by Berger (1979), in which religious belief itself becomes a private individualised concern. Furthermore, in Roman Catholic countries (such as Austria, France, the Irish Republic, Italy, Portugal and Spain), while the church continues to play a major role in the provision of care, increasingly secularised responses to the social needs associated with old age have been associated with growing industrialisation and urban life (Florea, 1979; Fleetwood, 1980; Huet and Fontaine, 1980; Sanidad y Seguridad, 1981; Bianchi, 1991).

What may be noticeable is the greater incidence of direct provision of welfare services for older people by churches in Roman Catholic and Orthodox countries (Amann, 1980a; Teperoglou, 1980; Carroll, 1991). For example, in Greece the Orthodox Church remains a main provider of welfare services other than pensions, and represents one end of the continuum of religious provision which is shared with some Catholic countries of Eastern Europe (Zarras, 1980; Hrynkiewicz *et al.*, 1991; Stathopoulos and Amera, 1992). However, this situation is predicted to alter as the effects of the changes during the later 1980s take effect, following which it is already possible for Greece to be characterised as having a high level of public ownership or control of care services (along with Italy and the UK), while Eastern Europe moves towards Western welfare models (Hunter, 1986; Dontas, 1987; Széman, 1992). Even though denominational services play a sizeable part in Germany and The Netherlands, they do so within the scope of state regulation and funding (Evers and Olk, 1991; Pijl, 1991). This pattern is following the one evident in Italy several decades ago, and in the UK towards the end of the nineteenth and during the early twentieth centuries, in which welfare responses to old age having their origins in religious organisations were gradually secularised, either within or under the control of the state (Hendricks and Hendricks, 1977, p. 281; Parry and Parry, 1979).

Across Europe, churches continue to play a part in the lives of many older people through an attachment to religious belief (however nominal). For example, in Greece, over 98 per cent of older people identify themselves as being members of the Orthodox Church (Teperoglou *et al.*, 1990). This is of some importance, because of the continuing church provision of services, amongst Roman Catholic and Protestant as well as Orthodox groups, even in the 'post-Christian' north (Evers and Olk, 1991; Pijl, 1991). There is also a widespread myth in Protestant countries that religious involvement increases in later life. This latter point is perhaps more easily dealt with by the evidence that religious belief and practice are more closely associated with generational patterns of social ideology prevalent among particular cohorts, than with ageing as such (for example, it was more widespread in the 1930s than the 1960s in the UK) (Wilson, 1976; Hendricks and Hendricks, 1977). The extent to which secularisation brings with it a less valued role for older people is more contentious.

Ageing and culture

Demographic explanations of the history of ageing suggest that because of the increase in the proportion of older people in industrialising Europe the evidence of ageing is more visible: there has been a greater presence of older people, especially among the dominant classes. From these demographic changes a different cultural dimension was introduced in Europe, and negative images of older people began to pervade literature and philosophy (Minois, 1989; Covey, 1991). This is not to say that a high status in old age is attached to rarity value (Cowgill, 1972, p. 9; Fennel *et al.*, 1988, p. 12). Rather, what emerged was a contradiction between the veneration of elderly people (triumphant survivors against the odds) and the despising of old age (loss of physical stature and social status) in which a distinction could be seen more clearly between the ideal and the reality of life for increasing numbers of people. The connection here with the changed economic role of surplus ex-worker appears to be strong, as these negative images stressed weakness and physical incapacity, and social as well as economic redundancy.

Redundancy has not necessarily been a unitary experience. Throughout Europe there are some social groups for whom retirement either is not inevitable or for whom the age of retirement is later than for others. Surprisingly, in the context of popular ideas about the loss of intellectual as well as physical capacity in ageing, politicians, judges, doctors and academics in many European countries retire later than their fellow citizens, or do not have a fixed formal retirement age. The same is true of artists and writers. In Italy, judges and academics may work until they are aged 70, compared to the general level of 60 or less; in Greece, senior civil servants retire at 65, compared to their junior colleagues at 62; in the former Yugoslavia, professors and judges retire five years later than other occupations; and in the UK it is only recently that the retirement age for university academics has been reduced to 65, and for doctors to 70. A debate about a formal age for the retirement of judges is taking place (albeit couched in terms of ageist assumptions) at the time of writing (Florea, 1980; Zarras, 1980; Rusica *et al.*, 1991). Politicians are subject to retirement by the electorate or by their own choice (at least in the liberal democracies); perhaps this is the most advantaged position of all. Although the public perception of the age of politicians may be affected by the high profile of a few individuals, in practice the average age of senior politicians in Europe has long been similar to that in other professional areas (de Beauvoir, 1977; Dontas *et al.*, 1991). Positively, such anomalies might appear to counter the cultural image, which has pervaded European culture for many centuries, of the inadequacy of the aged person. However, it should be recognised that these are privileged groups in terms of class, as well as being overwhelmingly male and white. In that sense they may be seen as the exceptions which prove the general rule.

De Beauvoir (1977) and Featherstone and Hepworth (1990) describe graphically how old age has been portrayed negatively to varying degrees in European theatre, art and literature from the time of Boccaccio and Chaucer onwards. Across Europe the old man was characterised as ridiculous, the old woman as pitiable, and both as physically disgusting. Within this uniformly discriminating gloss can be detected increasing evidence of gender divisions (Sontag, 1978). As Minois notes (1989, pp. 291–3), the rapid increase in the numbers of older people in the sixteenth century was related to improved hygiene in childbirth, especially among the aristocracy. In particular, more women survived, and by end of the sixteenth century the beginnings of greater life expectancy for women could be detected, which by the twentieth century has spread to all social classes. This is the period in which ideas such as the 'fading rose' and 'ugly duchess' gain credence, as the developing ideals of femininity and reality of old age came together, the latter confronting the former. It is in this period also that the persecution of older women as 'witches' reached its height. While it is only in the later part of the twentieth century that the sexuality of older people of either sex has come to be accepted as a positive aspect of life, judgements on ageing in women have been particularly harsh, reflecting both the wider social position of women and that those judging were, almost uniformly, men (Stearns, 1977, pp. 30–1; Covey, 1989). Ageing as the ending of reproductive capacity as opposed to diminished productive potential forms a double jeopardy for women, as both are devalued aspects of the life-cycle.

In short, it appears that to the concept of the 'exworker' we should add the 'ex-potential-producer-of-children', an ideological construct which ignores both the domestic labour of women and the value of older women to younger people as a source of assistance and advice. The 'wise elder' and 'triumphant survivor' has lived on in the domestic context, out of sight of the male-dominated world of politics, literature and science (Oakley, 1974; Rowbotham, 1974; Ehrenreich and English, 1979). The modern understanding of old age is therefore shaped by patriarchy as well as capitalism, and by the relationship between the two.

The stress on negative images in European culture is now possibly an overstatement, as many of the same writers have noted the advent of what could be described as a more positive note, with the development more recently of the capacity of elderly people in industrial society to exercise some power, based on the time and money available to them, hence forming a major economic grouping which is defined by consumption rather than production (Stearns, 1977; Fennell *et al.*, 1988). The limits to this more positive view are to be found in the social cleavages which have already been identified, of gender, sexuality, class and race, which will affect the incomes of older people, where they live, their wider social relationships and so on. We are faced with the reality that some older Europeans are increasingly well-off and able to enjoy travel and other 'leisure' activities while others remain in a similar state of poverty to previous generations. Old age is increasingly a divided stage of the life-cycle (Fogarty, 1986; Dieck, 1990; Teperoglou *et al.*, 1990; Pijl, 1991).

Another, more positive, development which can be identified is the rise of movements against the prejudicial and stereotyped views of old age in the 'Gray Panthers' and similar groups which promote the interests and needs of older people, although this is a phenomenon which has gained most ground in the USA where it originated (Elder, 1977; Hendricks and Hendricks, 1977; Phillipson, 1982; Bornat *et al.*, 1985; Kuhn, 1986). Part of their activity has been political and economic, in that they have campaigned for increased levels of pension for example, or against specific discriminations relating to old age. However, these movements are broadly cultural in so far as they promote positive images of ageing, of older people actively engaged in society and not merely passively dependent. This seeks to go beyond the power of older people as consumers, to emphasise the reciprocal relationship of older people to other social groups and of their integrity as full members of a society (Kuhn, 1986). However, the experience in Europe, exemplified by that in Germany and the UK, is that as a distinct movement the more militant tone of the Gray Panthers has not made such a big impact as in North America (Dieck, 1990).

A specific cultural institution that has developed in recent decades and which carries positive connotations of old age is the University of the Third Age movement (U3A), which has had an impact in France, Spain and the

UK (Huet and Fontaine, 1980; Dirección General JPS, 1981; Bornat *et al.*, 1985). This development, of an informal network of post-basic educational opportunities for older people, projects an image of old age as a continuation of adult life in which learning, growth and development do not have to give way to disengagement and withdrawal. However, because U3A is outside formal educational institutions and is run by older people it runs the risk that it might be considered as 'second best', good enough for elderly people but not taken seriously by educational policy-makers (Bornat *et al.*, 1985, p. 101). Yet, as Bornat *et al.* acknowledge, it puts the continuing education of adults on the social agenda. Other, more localised, consideration is being given to the availability of educational facilities to older people within mainstream provision, but this too is variable and subject to political and economic pressures which may set limits to the funding necessary to make such an opportunity available beyond those who are able to afford to pay for it (Lowy, 1979; Bornat *et al.*, 1985; Norton, 1992). The issue of education embodies the cultural contradiction of ageing, where there is an interplay of positive and negative factors. Such opportunities, while an indicator of the potential for changed attitudes, are at present available only to a relatively privileged minority (Laslett, 1989; Johnson and Falkingham, 1992).

The Family

In the foregoing discussion there has been frequent reference to connections between industrialisation, urbanisation and family structures. The modernisation thesis argues that advanced industrial societies, characterised by nuclear families, marginalise older people, isolating them and reducing their status (Cowgill and Holmes, 1972; Fischer, 1978). To what extent does the evidence from European countries support this view? How have developments in family structures and relationships affected older people?

There are two elements to these questions which it is necessary to disentangle: first, the extent to which there has been a growth of the nuclear family; second, the impact of any change on the roles and status of older people within the family. It is important to separate these issues because the possibility of structural change does not of itself determine the positive or negative value which might be perceived in any developments.

There is widespread support for the idea that the role and status of older people within the family has suffered a decline during the nineteenth and twentieth centuries, from that of a valued, central, even dominant member to that of someone who is at best marginal (even if regarded with affection), and at worst a burden. This was the conclusion reached by de Beauvoir (1977), while Tentori (1976) and Florea (1980) reported that in Italy family relationships between younger and older people were regarded as having become more stressed, with greater isolation from other family members experienced even where there is co-residence. However, de Beauvoir's conclusion was challenged by the observations of Huet and Fontaine regarding France (1980), and the assumption of a uniform decline in the status of older people has been questioned in other countries too. In Greece there is an ambivalent view, which sees the role and status of older people within the family as being in flux, declining in part (the loss of patriarchal authority, or some isolation caused by urbanisation and emigration) but strengthened in other respects (for example, in reciprocal exchanges such as the provision of child care to enable mothers to take paid employment in return for some other form of support) (Teperoglou, 1980; Teperoglou *et al.*, 1990; Pitsiou, 1986; Stathopoulos and Amera, 1992). This is similar to the pattern reported by Huet and Fontaine (1980). In the Irish Republic the integration of older people within families remains strong (although here too urbanisation and emigration has had an impact) (Fleetwood, 1980; Browne, 1990). In some Mediterranean countries there remains a strong sense of 'shame' in situations where a family is not able to provide a supportive role for aged members, and this may be buttressed by relative isolation in rural areas which keep relationships close because of the proximity of family members (Lisón-Tolosana, 1976; Nazareth, 1976; Pitsiou, 1986; Sant Cassia, 1992).

The evidence from northern Europe and Scandinavia, likewise, is that the social roles and status of older people within the family is changing, but that such changes do not amount to a clear rejection or devaluation. In the UK (as I noted in Chapter 2) there is a continuing culture of reciprocity, which is observable also in Germany and Scandinavia (Lowy, 1979; Sundström, 1986; Finch, 1989; Wærness, 1990). This may be set against the historical evidence of several centuries, demonstrated in a comparative study of Denmark and the UK, that relationships between younger and older adults have long been ambivalent, marked as much by opposing interests as by affection, where reciprocity breaks down because members of one or both generations do not act within the prevailing norms (Quadagno, 1982).

One particular facet of the 'decline of the elder' thesis is the view that co-residence has diminished – that older people are literally as well as socially excluded from the family. Contemporary data from urban France, Scandinavia and the UK which show that a majority of older people live alone or with only a partner only might be held to support this view

(Sundstrøm, 1986; Rhein, 1987; Bond, 1990; Wærness, 1990). However, this interpretation of the data is questionable (Victor, 1987). First, loss of role and status, even isolation, may be experienced even when there is co-residence. This is an important consideration, suggesting that it is not where or with whom one lives, but social relationships that are crucial. Second, in these countries co-residence was never a common pattern. However, in other countries, the lower incidence of coresidence has not resulted from a decline of the extended family: it was never the norm, except for some minority groups (see Bhalla and Blakemore, 1981; Barker, 1984). In Denmark, the separate residence of older people and their adult offspring was common in the rural agrarian era (Quadagno, 1982; Andersson, 1992). In Austria and Germany, the concept of 'intimacy at a distance' was coined to describe a long-standing pattern of social relationships in which it has long been usual for families to be located within close enough proximity for regular contact but not co-resident (Rosenmayr and Köckeis, 1963; Amann, 1980). This pattern of life is valued by older people as a means of maintaining independence (Rosenmayr, 1972). A similar pattern existed also in the UK over several centuries (Laslett, 1977).

Moreover, the separate residence of older people is only a modern phenomenon in some countries. In certain rural agrarian communities (such as parts of France, Greece, the Irish Republic, Italy, Poland, Portugal or Spain) co-residence has been normative, and may still continue where successive generations remain in the rural area (Lisón-Tolosana, 1976; Nazareth, 1976; Fleetwood, 1980; Zarras, 1980; Synak, 1987a).

Why, therefore, does the idea of the diminution of the extended family appear so widespread when there is evidence to support it only in some countries? Does it relate to changes in family care and support offered to older members? In fact, there is ample evidence from all countries in the EC and Scandinavia that family members are not only the first source of assistance when an elderly person has dependency needs, but are the sole or predominant source of care in the vast majority of instances, no matter how great a level of dependence is reached (Teperoglou, 1980; Sundstrøm, 1986; Finch, 1989; Parker, 1990; Wærness, 1990). Research findings in Norway show that the work of family members may be as much as eight times the level of formal care in terms of the number of care hours provided, while in Greece (where the traditional extended family does appear to be changing) there is a greater number of informal care recipients compared to all other forms of community care combined (Dontas, 1987; Wærness, 1990).

Not all family members actually provide care, no matter how extended the family may be. There was considerable research in the UK during the

1980s which demonstrated that women play an overwhelmingly large part in this work and that powerful sets of social mores operate to produce hierarchies of obligation to care, with gender and consanguinity the most powerful factors (Finch and Groves, 1980; Qureshi and Walker, 1989). However, family care is not only intergenerational: in the UK as many as 90 per cent of married elderly people receive care from their partners (Wenger, 1984). Moreover, when men provide care it is most likely to be for a spouse, suggesting that most male carers are likely to be older (Evandrou *et al.*, 1986). Similar patterns in the distribution of family care can be seen in Scandinavia, and in other EC countries (Wærness, 1990; Jani-Le Bris, 1992). In practice, therefore, the range of key relationships which constitute 'the family' is likely to be quite small and to have very clear boundaries despite varying between individual instances, although too restrictive a definition is neither useful nor appropriate (Qureshi and Walker, 1989).

A more plausible explanation for the pervasiveness of the idea that older people have lost a valued position within the pattern of family relationships may be adduced from a consideration of the specific issue of loneliness. As noted on page 51, Shanas *et al.* (1968), in their formative study, showed that a large proportion of older people in Denmark, the UK and the USA assessed family networks in comparison to the lives of their younger relatives, to their own lives slightly earlier, and to their ideological images of previous generations. In more recent studies, particularly those in areas with a strong traditional background of large extended families, there is a high level of self-reported loneliness by older people. In Greece and Poland, for example, some studies have shown that this level may exceed the proportions of older people living alone or with an elderly partner (Synak, 1987b; Jylhä and Jokela, 1990). It may be greater also than the proportion who reported not being visited by a family member during the previous day (that is, some people who have family contact report themselves as being lonely) (Pitsiou, 1986; Dontas, 1987; Jylhä and Jokela, 1990). Jylhä and Jokela (1990, p. 310) identify the culturally normative component of these views: it is not the fact of social contact *per se* that is an appropriate yardstick of loneliness, but the range of contacts compared to the older person's social values. They point out that in Greek there is no exact translation of the English word 'privacy', and in such a culture a small amount of contacts may not feel as significant in comparison to perceptions in the more individualistic Anglo-Saxon world. To render the English word 'privacy' in Greek is problematic, as a distinction is made in Greek between the equivalent of either 'loneliness' and 'isolation' on the one hand or else 'peace' and 'tranquillity' on the other, which carry very different connotations in Greek as well as English (Triantafillou and Mestheneos, 1990). In this cultural context the gap between reality and ideal may generate a sense of dissatisfaction or loss. Indeed, complaints about the phenomenon of loneliness in old age have a long history in Europe (Minois, 1989).

Yet such an explanation would not account for the similar sense of change throughout the Anglo-Saxon world. Critics of the modernisation theory of family relationships have pointed to socioeconomic accounts of prestige in old age in pre-industrial society, and in the control by parents over land and other forms of wealth, even in relatively poor families (Quadagno, 1982; MacFarlane, 1986). This has certainly diminished with industrialisation, just as the Mediterranean family network has actually become smaller. However, the prestige deriving from the power associated with even limited wealth produces conflict as much as respect, so it is more probable that any continuing sense of lost status or value in old age reflects other changes.

In both social anthropology and sociology the term 'golden age' has been used to describe an ideological process in which assumptions that things 'were better in the past' or 'will get better in the future' plays an almost autonomous part in the formation of both public and private think-ing (Pearson, 1975). It is a pertinent observation in the context of this dis-cussion that such golden ages tend to stand as a criticism of the present. Yet why should a golden view of ageing have gained such credence in the latter part of the twentieth century? Two factors are apparent. First, the evidence in the 1960s that poverty in Europe had not been overcome in the post-war reconstruction, and that the economic boom particular affected older people (Townsend and Wedderburn, 1965; de Beauvoir, 1977; Townsend, 1979). Because of their social situation large numbers of older people did not share in the growing prosperity of the industrialised countries. In this sense, the 'rediscovery of poverty' was a revisiting of class and other social divisions, recognising that older people are not a monolithic group. Second, as the economic boom began to falter in the late 1960s and early 1970s the implications for welfare-state economics was a deepening crisis which has resulted in the breakdown of consensus about the scale and structure of welfare (O'Connor, 1973; Guillemard, 1983; Mishra, 1984). A similar process is taking place in eastern Europe (Boeri, 1993). Given the demographic changes which have meant that older people are the main users of social welfare services, to reduce the level of state spending on these services required a reconstruction of social ideology to promote private solutions to the public problem of welfare provision. An emphasis on 'the family', as if this were not already the main source of support and care for older people, has therefore emerged in European social policy (Henrard, 1991; Jack, 1991). Even in Scandinavian countries, where consensus about the welfare state has been most entrenched, a reappraisal and refocusing of emphasis towards the family has taken place (Daatland, 1992).

In this way, the relationship between older people and the family is a political issue, and the continuing force of ideas about the loss of role and status of old age within the family has to be seen in this context. Although the modernisation thesis which supports this view was originally developed in relation to historical material dating back two hundred years, its articulation occurred at a juncture where the optimism of social policy reform was being challenged. It is around the concept of 'the family' that ideas about modernisation and demographic change have been brought together to legitimate the restructuring of the welfare state. The place of older people within the family is a major component of these changes.

So in this sense it is not the family which has abandoned older people but rather that the significance of the family for older people has been subject to shifting perception and debate, fuelled by other social and political changes. The family remains a major institution in Europe for older people as well as for other members. I will return in later chapters to the pressures on the family as a source of care in contemporary circumstances, and its relationship to specific types of formal care which have developed.

The European History of Ageing

This brief overview of historical factors has sought to identify threads in the construction of ageing in Europe through economic, cultural and social forces. The emerging picture is one of diversity. What it means to be old, how that part of life is moulded and experienced, differs according to the economic background of both a country and an individual, where the older person lives (in a city or the countryside), the religious and other ideological background of a country, and how family relationships are structured. There are common threads running across countries, which are then divided by other issues. Within each country, and also between older people themselves there are social divisions of class, gender, race and ethnicity, as well as regional differences.

To this extent it is not possible to talk of a single history or culture of ageing in Europe, but rather of a series of histories which overlap. In Chapter 2 I characterised the difference between Greece and the UK as one of polarisation with respect to each of these factors. However, in this chapter the interconnections between different economic and cultural aspects of ageing have been shown to cluster European countries differently according to the specific issue under discussion. It is for this reason that I have not sought to develop a single schema incorporating all relevant factors; nor has it been possible to include reference to all countries in each point. Those countries which differ in relation to industrialisation or urban life may have similarities with respect to retirement policies, or to family structures, and so on. Therefore we do not have a straightforward polarity, but a complex set of divisions, between north and south, east and west, EC and non-EC, urban and rural, industrial and agrarian. Countries themselves will be divided regionally. There is no single causal linkage which would enable countries to be typified with respect to levels of pension, retirement age, levels of formal care, who provides formal care and so on. How the modern history or culture of ageing in Europe is characterised will depend on the particular aspect of ageing under scrutiny and the location of our observations.

The significance of this multidimensional understanding of the social construction of ageing will be developed further in later chapters, in a consideration of policies and professional practices concerning ageing and the needs of older people. Before that, I want to examine in more detail contemporary issues surrounding the ambivalence about old age and older people which, as we have seen, runs through European society and which shapes both our understanding of and our responses to old age.

4

Respect and Abuse

Images of Old Age

Social values

Analysis and discussion of the social roles and status of older people in Europe, as well as North America and Australasia, in recent years have been dominated by a concern about the extent to which ageing and older people are positively valued. As we have already seen, one strand of social gerontology has developed in response to perceptions of the loss of positive value, in the formulation of the modernisation theory (Cowgill and Holmes, 1972; Fischer, 1978; Gruman, 1978). Many more gerontologists, other professionals and older people themselves are critical of the phenomenon of *ageism*; that is, discrimination between people on grounds of age when this is not a relevant issue (Phillipson, 1982; Fogarty, 1986; Itzin, 1986; Walker, 1986b; Featherstone and Hepworth, 1990). Such ideas about ageing and older people not only influence the thoughts and actions of scientists, politicians and professionals but also pervade the whole of society, being reflected in everyday language. As such, the perception and experience of ageing is embedded in an array of social values, within which the identities of individuals and groups are structured and maintained (Goffman, 1971).

Of particular interest in recent years has been the identification of *elder abuse*; that is, the harming, exploitation or intimidation of an elderly person in which the old age of the victim is a key element of the harm which is perpetrated (for example, through vulnerability arising from a dependency relationship) (Eastman, 1984; Glendenning, 1993; Penhale, 1993). Concern has focused in particular on carers, whether 'formal' (such as a professional) or 'informal' (such as a family member) (Dieck, 1987; Council of Europe, 1992; Pritchard, 1992; Stathopoulos and Amera, 1992). The emergence of this issue would appear to be the culmination of the efforts to raise the profile of ageing in the professional and public spheres,

in which private difficulties have been constructed as social problems
(Leroux and Petrunik, 1990; Phillipson and Biggs, 1992).

It is against this background that I want to consider the value component
of ageing in European countries and to explore questions about the extent
to which old age and older people are esteemed or denigrated, respected or
abused. This discussion will focus not only on the contemporary identification of 'elder abuse' but also on the wider value context within which
this phenomenon is to be understood. In particular, the extent to which
European societies are ageist, in their construction of and response to old
age, must form a basis for any discussion of the actions of specific groups
or individuals (Gruman, 1978). So first of all I want to look in more depth
at negative social images of ageing and some examples of the phenomenon
of ageism.

Origins of negative social images

Whether it is in literature, philosophy or science, the individuality of the
older person is subsumed within the search for generalised types, theories or
laws. What it means to be old becomes stereotyped to some degree, and the
wide variety between different older people is lost. The common theme
which can be identified within European thought about old age over many
centuries is that of decline, in which a loss of physical and intellectual
capacity in ageing is matched by a reduction of social status. In the work of
both de Beauvoir (1977) and Minois (1989) the extent of these negative
images clearly outweighs the corresponding positive ascriptions of value,
honour, wisdom and so on. As Minois argues, the association between physical and social decline has often been very strong, so that as long as older
people retained their capacities they would be regarded as part of the more
general 'adult' population. This is epitomised in the early Scandinavian
literature, in which the prestige of older men is honoured in terms of their
former exploits, while further south in Frankish culture the 'white beard'
symbolised the warriors who had 'lost nothing of their strength and daring'
and for whom age conferred 'prestige, experience and wisdom' (Minois,
1989, p. 190). In Scandinavia, women too were honoured in this way, sometimes exercising matriarchal rule (p. 191). Yet, as Minois makes clear,
honour had to be maintained against infirmity; failure to do this could lead
to pitiable decline, and he records numerous literary examples of old
warriors actively seeking death to avoid such an end (for example, by
undertaking hazardous sea voyages).

As de Beauvoir and Minois agree, by the Middle Ages old age had
become a stage in the life-cycle that had much less value, because for most

people it had no meaning apart from decrepitude. Retirement is a product of modern industrial capitalism, and in the Middle Ages one worked until one died or was too infirm to continue (Minois, 1989, p. 207). In such a context the idea of old age became indissolubly bound up with loss of social participation. Medieval theories and scientific laws, such as the reworking of classical 'ages of man' (*sic*) concepts, were formulations which represented attempts to make sense of these social developments (Gruman, 1978). As an image, the idea of ageing as a series of distinct stages feeds into the concept of retirement in such a way that it emphasises the centuries-old prejudice that lies behind the notion that at a certain age one should expect to take on a less active social role.

In cultures outside Europe also, old people appear to have been typified as a burden as frequently as they have been seen as a benefit, if not more so (Silverman and Maxwell, 1982; Victor, 1985). Silverman and Maxwell (1982, pp. 66–7) recorded active killing or abandonment of elderly people in twenty out of ninety-six pre-industrial societies, and a more passive neglect or low status in more than half of the remainder. The earlier work of Simmons (1945) had also shown a large minority (eighteen out of thirty-nine) of pre-industrial societies abandoning or killing dependent elderly people. The different patterns of active rejection could include ritual killing in ceremonial or festive form, or else abandonment sanctioned by group norms; sometimes both patterns might occur in the same society (Victor, 1987). The older person often appears to have been expected to take part willingly in the arrangement of their own death, and some anthropological evidence includes folk tales which seem to play a part in supporting these practices, contrasting the honour of acceptance with the ignominy of resistance (de Beauvoir, 1977, pp. 62–3).

Anthropological evidence suggests that such types of euthanasia were most usually found among nomadic or semi-nomadic hunters rather than in settled agricultural societies (Silverman and Maxwell, 1982). Explanations of this phenomenon rest largely on the necessity in such cultures for adults to be able to contribute to economic activity (including the collection or preparation of food) and to be mobile so as not to threaten group survival. Thus it is not chronological age to which these reports refer but rather to infirmity associated with age. In those settled societies where such practices have been described there has been widespread poverty which would have had similar implications for the extent to which the 'productivity' of older people might contribute to images of the aged person as 'a burden' (de Beauvoir, 1977). At the same time there are several recorded instances of very poor nomadic societies in which older people were highly venerated and not subjected to euthanasia. In Chapter 2 I considered Victor's summary of the factors which affect the status of older people, and noted that productivity might also include usefulness to the preservation of culture (including religion and law), and that this factor is held to explain such differences. So Europe can be seen within a global continuum of social responses to old age; it does not represent an extreme cultural example.

In modern European society, as we have seen in Chapter 3, older age has become defined in terms of retirement from employment. As such it is possible to conclude that we are the inheritors of negative images of ageing from pre-industrial societies, either figuratively or in reality. While the literal killing of elderly people has not taken place formally in European cultures for many centuries, the social 'mortifications' deriving from a variety of age-related practices may be said to have taken its place. The chief of these in the modern era is compulsory retirement, associated as it is with the relatively high levels of poverty among older people (Walker, 1981; Guillemard, 1983). However, this is only one expression of a wider understanding of 'natural' biological ageing, in which physical decline continues to be associated powerfully with assumptions about intellectual capacity and social skills. It is reflected also in art and litera-ture, in common-sense thinking about sexuality and social relationships, in humour, and even in personal experiences of the ageing process (ISPA, 1976; Victor, 1987; Featherstone and Hepworth, 1990; Covey, 1989 and 1991).

Yet at the same time there are several important points on which the social construction of old age in modern Europe does not derive from past denigrations:

1. Modern Europe, for the most part, is less poor than in previous eras, and so the economic implications of maintaining those who are no longer required or allowed to work is less of an issue; the extent to which wealth is shared with those who have not taken part in its immediate production is a political choice and not a pragmatic expedient for survival;

2. With markedly increased numbers of older people, the idea of older people as a minority becomes questionable; moreover, the vast major-ity of adults of working age will look forward to a long retirement rather than working up to their death, so the social benefit of having this status constructed as a desirable goal is enhanced; and

3. The privatised nuclear model of the family which has developed under industrial capitalism, while in some sense causing part of the loss of

social status for older people, at the same time provides a basis for an adapted role which can give meaning to the lives of many older people as well as forming a major source of direct care and support when this is necessary.

In short, the means, motive and opportunity exist for the negative aspects of the social status of older people to be mitigated or challenged.

Yet, as we have already noted, the sense of 'burden' in other times and places was not associated in a direct way with chronological ageing as is compulsory retirement, but rather with dependence arising from infirmity or senescence. This image, sketched out in previous generations and other cultures, has a contemporary flavour in so far as the responsibility for providing direct care to older people with dependency needs falls disproportionately on certain people (see the discussion in Chapter 3 regarding hierarchies of social obligation). Women who are close relatives of an older person with care needs is highlighted here. They may well feel the impact of providing care in lost work opportunities and low income, social isolation, and physical and emotional strain (Finch and Groves, 1982; Ungerson, 1987; Qureshi and Walker, 1989; Wærness, 1990). The 'burden' which is described in this research literature is comparable to the sense of encumbrance described in preindustrial societies; as with preindustrial societies it is a social construction, although one which revolves around different cultural expectations, family structures and patterns of employment. In this way dependence in old age is constructed in modern society so that the interests of family members are at risk of being set in conflict, and both the elderly person and the carer may become trapped as the latter shares the 'social death' of the former. This contrasts with the ideal of mutual exchange (Steinmetz, 1988; Finch, 1989; Pitkeathley, 1989). Expressions of concern for the needs of carers may then take on unintended tones of devaluing the dependent elderly people (Morris, 1992).

A digression on ageing as experience

The extent to which we experience ourselves to be 'ageing' or 'old' is set in the context of expectations which derive from our social *milieu*. If perceptions of ageing as loss and decrepitude are reinforced routinely then we are likely to be faced with a dissonance between our objective and subjective experience. The English author J. B. Priestley described graphically a sharp break between how one feels and how one looks, as if one was forced to put on the attributes of age while remaining the same youthful person inside: it was, he felt, as if he had been forced to assume a false identity, that of an 'old man' (quoted in Featherstone and Hepworth, 1990). As Featherstone and Hepworth (1990, p. 253) point out, the language which surrounds old age and older people tends not to provide the materials with which to construct a positive identity. Each language has a store of denigrations for old age, and some expressions which may appear affectionate or jocular can also be patronising (for example, by using diminutives such as 'grannie'). At times it may be possible to reclaim some of these concepts as a matter of pride, such as the 'Gray Panthers', but for the most part 'wrinkly' (currently fashionable in the English speaking world), 'fogey' and so on do not lend themselves to positive connotations, even if we do agree that there is a need to construct more positive views (in order to promote mental health in older people, for example) (Dittman-Kohli, 1990). Epithets such as 'senile' and 'geriatric' may lend an air of acceptability based on popular conceptions of science, but these terms are widely misused in popular language. They refer to a physical and intellectual condition and a branch of medicine respectively but have come simply to mean 'old' and so add to the stock of derogatory words by which older people may be marginalised (Norman, 1987).

Negative self-images of ageing are also maintained by powerful economic interests. The profits of the cosmetics industry, largely European-based, depend in part on providing disguises for the effects of normal biological ageing of the skin and hair. As we have just noted, these are some of the attributes which form the basis of denigratory language. The advertising which supports the sales of cosmetics is therefore both a response to and a reinforcer of the more general social stereotypes of ageing. Ageism here also interweaves with sexism, as older women are subjected to the pressure of needing to 'look good' to a greater extent than are men (Sontag, 1978). However, for both sexes there is a relationship between the stereotypes of ageing and the extent to which we are able to maintain a positive identity. Wealth may provide greater access to the remedy, but the problem is the same, namely the internalisation of negative images of ageing which serve economic interests.

Ageism as image

All older people are to some extent oppressed by ageism. Judgements are made about the social worth of the older person in terms of their chronological age, and negative attributes may be assigned, even by older people themselves, either which are not appropriate to an individual or which are misconstrued. For example, in the UK approximately two-thirds of disabled people are over 60 years of age but only approximately half the people in this age group have a disability; and of the latter most are aged over 80 years (OPCS, 1988). The incidence of disability is comparable across several countries including Denmark, France, Germany, Italy and The Netherlands, and yet images of ageing often draw on disability or dependence as if this defined the majority experience of old age (Featherstone and Hepworth, 1990; Henrard, 1991; Anderson, 1992; Jani-Le Bris, 1992). Moreover, having a disability does not of itself affect an individual's capacity to engage in ordinary social life: the exclusion of disabled people from mainstream life is produced through discriminatory social relationships and actions (Oliver, 1990). Disability is closely related to discrimination against older people: that is, to ageism. Both are means of exclusion because disabled people and older people do not 'conform' to the social norm of the younger physically able-bodied person. Similarly, the so-called 'demographic crisis' of the numbers of older people in European society is partially constructed around the idea that older people generally are a burden (ISPA, 1976; Gruman, 1978; de Jouvenal, 1988; Coleman and Bond, 1990; Jack, 1991; Pitaud *et al.*, 1991).

Another form of ageism can be seen in the overwhelming interest of professionals and politicians in the needs of older people compared to their potential contribution to society (Fogarty, 1986; Fennell *et al.*, 1988). This emphasis interacts with the wider social constructions to reinforce negative images (such as 'old age equals dependence') while at the same time being part of the expression of social concern for needy groups of older people. In this sense ageism is part of a wider contradiction, in which the older person is both a worthy recipient of social concern and at the same time an unproductive absorber of social wealth (Gruman, 1978; Pitaud *et al.*, 1991).

It is in the contradictions of ageism that the foundations for the experience of respect and abuse of older people are laid. The gaps between expressions of the worthiness of older people on the one hand and the problems created by the social organisation of responses to the 'burden' of old age on the other are wider than is usually recognised in public policy. The consequence is that expectations about respect for older people are maintained or promoted at the same time as circumstances undermine opportunities to act on this ideology. Where outcomes fail to match the ideal they tend to be seen as the problem of individuals and where they involve carers may increasingly be characterised as 'elder abuse'.

Elder Abuse

What is 'elder abuse'?

The identification of a distinct phenomenon concerning the harming of elderly people by their carers is recent, even though such events may not be (Steinmetz, 1988). Beginning in North America, there has been a growing concern among professionals and social scientists that a large number of older people are harmed by family members or others who provide care for them. 'Elder abuse' has been defined as 'the systematic maltreatment, physical, emotional or financial, of an elderly person by a care-giving relative', although it is recognised that there is a lack of consensus about what might actually constitute maltreatment (Eastman, 1984, pp. 23–4). In a review of definitions used in the USA, Breckman and Adelman (1988) distinguish between intentional and unintentional neglect or mistreatment of an older person by a care-giver or other family member, as well as identifying the separate issue of self-harm or neglect by older people (whether intentional or not). Within this framework, mistreatment may involve domestic violence, but this is not necessary for actions to be seen as abusive. Moreover, neglect on the part of a carer also may be seen as abusive, such as failing to provide food or warmth or to seek appropriate medical assistance. In some studies, for example Dieck (1987) and Kurrle *et al.* (1991), a clear distinction is made between 'abuse', which is reserved for active harming, and 'neglect', which is passive. In a small proportion of instances abuse may take the form of rejection, either abandoning a relative or refusing to accept their return from hospital (de Beauvoir, 1977; Eastman, 1984; Steinmetz, 1988; Council of Europe, 1992).

What is apparent from these formulations is that for the most part the phenomenon of 'elder abuse' has been identified in the informal, everyday contexts of family care. Even where structural explanations are given for the origins of people's actions, or abuse is identified in professional contexts (such as hospitals or residential care), mistreatment and neglect are constructed as individual, interpersonal problems.

The individualisation of 'elder abuse' can be seen partly as a reflection of general social ideologies of the family (as discussed above) and partly as the outcome of public policy which 'residualises' welfare provision (to which I will return below). That is, families are faced with a context in which they are expected to provide the direct care of older people with high levels of dependency needs (whether of physical frailty or mental infirmity) but which at the same time is not conducive to the consequences of the caring role (Ungerson, 1987; Steinmetz, 1988; Pitkeathley, 1989; Wærness,

1990). The social isolation and poverty experienced by carers may also be compounded by the direct physical and mental effort in providing the care, lifting the older person, performing intimate care tasks (often for a parent or partner), as well as the more mundane routine domestic work. In such circumstances the carer may experience the role as a burden, and transfer this to the older person psychologically (through the emotional and other interpersonal aspects of the relationship) or physically (by withholding care or by direct ill-treatment) (Eastman, 1984; Stang, 1986; Steinmetz, 1988).

A major source of stress leading to abuse by a family carer has been identified as a conflict of role expectation, in which well-established notions of seniority (the parent and the child is the most usual example) are confounded by increased dependency. This derives from the power of 'childhood' as the culturally normative model of dependence. When dependence becomes profound the impact may go beyond simple role reversal, and become a generational inversion which challenges the prior social and psychological basis of relationships (Foulke, 1980, quoted in Steinmetz, 1988, pp. 47–9).

Breckman and Adelman (1988, p. 30) draw attention to a further distinction, in that 'elder abuse' may not be intergenerational but be between spouses. They argue that it is necessary also to understand whether this is of recent origin or a life-long pattern, in order to be able to think about how policy-makers and professionals might respond. Garland (1990, p. 128) quotes the example of a mentally frail woman caring for her physically disabled partner in a way which unintentionally put him at risk of harm: should this be construed as 'elder abuse'? Similarly, what of the man who in older age assaults his partner, but has done so for fifty years? It may be more appropriate to see the former as a problem of how care and support might be provided to the couple, while the latter is more accurately seen as domestic violence in which age is a secondary issue, if an issue at all (Breckman and Adelman, 1988; Callahan, 1988; Steinmetz, 1988; Leroux and Petrunik, 1990). Both these constructions avoid the problem of ageism, without denying the extent to which some mistreatment or violence may arise from age- related circumstances.

A further complication in the definition of abuse can arise in situations either where the dependent older person is an abuser, or else mistreatment is mutual (Eastman, 1984; Marin, 1992). Again, it may be that the origin of the mistreatment is in increased dependency or it may not (Kurrle *et al.*, 1991). Situations may arise where, for example, a parent who has ill-treated a child now depends on that person for care but continues the ill-treatment, or else the carer now has the opportunity for reprisal, or both. In each of these possibilities age is only one factor among many, and then only in so far as it is associated with an increase in frailty (physical or mental). In such situations the term 'elder abuse' may appear to absolve the older person of responsibility for their own actions, a response which would in itself be ageist. Therefore, setting such events within the broader category of domestic and family relationships is more appropriate.

Ungerson's distinction between caring *about* and caring *for* is useful here to draw a line between the emotional commitment to older family members which is socially valued (caring about) and the provision of direct domestic labour (caring for), which in European society become intertwined (Ungerson, 1983). We show that we care *about* by caring *for*, although the onus does not fall equally within the family, being gender-divided, as we have seen above. In such a situation someone who does not perform caring *for* sufficiently well is seen to be not caring *about*. Even though caring labour may be (or come to be) performed out of a sense of duty and obligation rather than an emotional commitment, or be an expression of genuine commitment beyond the capacity of the carer, both the individual and the wider society may regard ill-treatment as a failure in the exercise of caring responsibilities. This will be seen as a problem at the personal level, to the point where individual culpability will be attached. However, even the intentional inflicting of violence on the older person can be seen as one end of a continuum rather than as a separate category of action, because the common elements to each of the forms of 'elder abuse' which have been identified are a conflict between the social pressures on families to provide care, the extent of support offered to families, the physical and emotional demands of providing care, and the complexities of family relationships.

The emergence of 'elder abuse'

'Elder abuse' as such is not a new phenomenon. An example quoted from a district nurse who worked in an English village in the 1920s highlights this:

> Old people were not taken care of. This is another thing which people like to think now, that grandfathers and grandmothers had an honoured place in the cottage. In fact, when they got old they were just neglected, pushed away into corners. I even found them in cupboards! Even in fairly clean and respectable houses you often found an old man or woman shoved out of sight in a dark niche. (Blythe, 1972, p. 231)

Although this is only one person's recollection, it seems unlikely that these responses to old age were confined to one village, or even to England alone. This is borne out by de Beauvoir's (1977, p. 277) detailed discussion of France in which it is noted that poverty and poor housing exacerbate the situation. The complexities of care, which may result in instances of neglect or abuse, do not appear to have changed very much over several centuries, as patterns of family life have fluctuated rather than changing dramatically (Laslett, 1977; Fennell *et al.*, 1988). Similar patterns are evident in the more extensive North American literature (Steinmetz, 1988; Wolf and Pillemer, 1989; Leroux and Petrunik, 1990).

Yet the emergence of 'elder abuse' has not only happened at a time when there are increased pressures against individuals caring for older family members, but also against the background of the development across Europe of policies which emphasises the family as the locus of caring (albeit to varying degrees in different countries) (Henrard, 1991; Council of Europe, 1992). The possibility that family members may not be able to meet the expectations embodied in policy is an underlying dimension which enables professional concern for the safety of individuals to be heard in a particular way: that is, as a problem requiring professional intervention. The 'discovery' of 'elder abuse' may be said therefore to have taken place as a response not to a sudden exposure of what has been happening over a long period but to changes in thought within professional and political groups concerned about the welfare of older people, which have enabled the perception of the phenomenon to develop in these terms (Leroux and Petrunik, 1990).

Professional abuse?

The classification of neglect or ill-treatment of older people who are in need of care as 'abuse' has tended to focus on individuals within families, pathologising actions which may be grounded in contradictory social circumstances (Council of Europe, 1992). This approach has demonstrated that such violence or neglect takes place in all European countries, and charts its incidence at varying levels. However, this focus has tended to distract attention from the possibility of similar actions being undertaken by formal professional carers at an individual level (Tornstam, 1989), or else the systematic neglect or ill-treatment by organisational structures and social policies of older people as a group.

For example, Phillipson (1982), Walker (1986a) and Laczko (1990) have pointed to the continuing widespread poverty experienced by older people which is a direct consequence of social security policies. Laczko (1990) concluded that while poverty among older people generally is lower than it was twenty years ago and is variable across the EC, it is still relatively high. Using 'poverty line' measures, studies suggest that poverty is experienced by between 17.5 per cent and 25 per cent in Belgium, France, Italy, The Netherlands and the UK (Fogarty, 1986; Laczko, 1990). Mean average pensions are at a replacement rate for earnings of 60 per cent in most EC countries, although they vary from 46 per cent (UK) to 90 per cent (The Netherlands) (Laczko, 1990). Moreover, poverty among older people is increasing in Denmark, Italy, The Netherlands and Portugal, although it is decreasing in all other EC countries (and quite markedly in Belgium, the Irish Republic and France) (Eurostat, 1990). It may reasonably be asked, however, if societies which create or perpetuate poverty among some citizens on the grounds of their age can be said to be engaged in structural neglect or ill-treatment. In consumer-orientated society disposable resources are as much a basis of social power as the ownership of property: poverty is socially disempowering as well as personally demeaning. It is known also that poverty is greater, proportionately, among women and members of ethnic minorities and this compounds the issue, linking ageism with sexism and racism (Walker, 1987). Sweden and Norway are the possible exceptions in Europe, at least as regards the position of women (Sheppard and Mullins, 1989; Wærness, 1990).

Some other disadvantages and discriminations faced by older people arise from poverty or low income. Low-standard housing, inadequate food and warmth, and isolation resulting from the lack of funds to pay for transport are some of the consequences of low income. The latter aspect can be particularly important where someone has a physical disability. Each of these factors emphasises low social status. Although such factors affect a minority of older people, because they arise from the level of pensions provision do so on the grounds of age and so are ageist.

Health and welfare professions too are implicated in discrimination against older people. In medicine, nursing, the remedial therapies and social work, services for older people are frequently regarded as being of lower status, and may attract less qualified staff (Chandler *et al.*, 1986; Howe, 1986; Triantafillou *et al.*, 1986; Biggs, 1989; Dieck, 1990). The fully qualified professionals who do chose to work in this area are likely to have made the choice for reasons other than professional prestige. Endemic in these professions are stereotypical attitudes towards older people, seeing them as requiring less skilful help or as being less capable of achieving the changes which indicate a successful outcome. There are some variations in appropriate professional responds to older people: biological ageing does affect the capacity of the human body to heal after disease or injury, for example. However, what I am arguing is that where in other groups of service users such 'obstacles' to the professional process would be seen as worthy challenges, among elderly people the image of a 'burden' is reproduced. For example, in most European countries the medical speciality of geriatrics is either non-existent or has only recently been developed, although this may be set against the specialist interest of some general medical practitioners (Hunter, 1986). However, other studies have elicited negative views of older people, in which they are seen to be problematic because they do not provide professional variety or interest (Howe, 1986; Dieck, 1990; Triantafillou and Mestheneos, 1990).

Biggs (1989) analyses professional responses to work with older people in relation to three factors, which he argues are interconnected. First, most professionals approach older people with an attitude formed from a mixture of stereotypes (derived from the society in which they live and work) and personal experiences (which will include problems and fears), and under this circumstances it may be difficult to maintain a positive perception of the people for whom one is working. Second, although professionals exercise power over older people, they are unlikely themselves to be in a relatively powerful position *vis-à-vis* their profession or employing agency. Their marginal status reflects that of their service user constituency. So, third, there is likely to be a higher degree of conformity to the projects of the service agencies than to those of older people themselves. These factors serve to explain the denigratory remarks noted above as part of a tendency to individualise the origins of marginalisation as a trait of older people rather than by locating them in social structures and cultural values. The consequence can be that older people are coerced into situations they do not want, given low standards of service, and on occasion actually ill-treated (Eastman, 1984; Marin, 1992). Each of these outcomes may be seen to be a form of professional 'elder abuse'. Where professionals actually harm older people there is a tendency to ascribe individualised explanations, whether of the professional or of the specific institution or agency. Society is 'scandalised' when individual nurses or social workers ill-treat an elderly service user, but the way in which the organisation of institutional care may promote such incidents is often ignored (Miller and Gwynne, 1972; Martin, 1984; Marin, 1992). I will return to this issue in Chapter 6.

Another way in which professionals (as well as others) can denigrate older people is by patronising them, either through forms of social relationship which are not age appropriate (infantilising) or the ambiguous use of diminutives, which in some cultures might normally convey respect but may also be used to denigrate an older person. For example, Triantafillou and Mestheneos (1990, p. 61) note such a use of the terms 'grandad' (*papou*) or 'grandma' (*yiayia*) amongst nurses and care workers in Greece. A similar tone is set by the use of first names for adults who may not have wished to be addressed in a familiar fashion or where it is not mutual (in contrast, see Allen *et al.*, 1992, p. 197), and even some services which are highly thought of by older people may carry unintentionally infantilising titles (such as 'fostering' to describe substitute family care) (Hugman, 1982). Among some paid helpers this can be an unconscious reflection of the low social status of the dependent older person, as with unqualified care workers who overtly are intending to convey warmth (again, care as a mix of labour and love). With others, such as qualified professionals, it is part of the social power which they exercise routinely through the use of language (Fairclough, 1989; Hugman, 1991). Evers (1981) draws attention to the gendered nature of these professional attitudes, in which dependency is seen as being less demeaning for a man than a woman, because of cultural expectations about women's capacity to cope with self-care. However, in all situations, the marginal and powerless position of those people who depend on others for daily care is emphasised, and their adult status is remodelled into one which more closely resembles infancy. There are similarities with the phenomenon of generational inversion discussed above, and European culture still lacks a more appropriate model for dependency in adulthood than that which is derived from childhood (Hugman, 1982).

In diverse ways older people may be 'abused' by social policies, organisational structures and professional practices. As I have noted above, there is a tendency by individual professionals and policy-makers as well as a system bias towards the pathologising of individuals, looking either externally to policies and practices or else defining instances of actual ill-treatment as individual exceptions. In part this is a consequence of the social construction of professions, a trained incapacity to see beyond 'the case' (Mills, 1956); in part, however, it is constructed around the denigration and powerlessness of older people as a social group. In the next section of this chapter I want to examine some of the recent professional and policy responses which have been formulated.

The ambiguity of responses to 'elder abuse'

Although the mistreatment of older people by carers has been the subject of research and professional intervention for some time, at a policy level it has only recently become an identified issue (Council of Europe, 1992). In the UK a national report has noted a 'lack of priority in formulating policies both national and local about elder abuse' (Social Services

Inspectorate, 1992, p. 19). The UK report lists the elements of a policy as including a definition of the problem, its location in the wider social context, including the multiracial nature of the UK, and the resources for a response including professional skills and organisational structures. In Germany, Dieck (1987) has noted that there has been a reluctance to address the issue, although recent reports have begun this process (Vierter Familienbericht, 1986). Elsewhere in Europe policy is still at the stage of problem recognition (Council of Europe, 1992).

Problem definition may be said to be the crucial component of policy responses to 'elder abuse', because of the variety of ways in which the same events can be defined. The perception of a distinct social phenomenon which can be termed 'elder abuse' has come to Europe from the USA, by way of the UK (because theoretical and empirical work has been published mainly in English), and so has brought with it many American assumptions, and these have been influential in other countries such as Australia and Canada (Eastman, 1984; Stang, 1986; Dieck, 1987; Leroux and Petrunik, 1990; Kurrle *et al.*, 1991; Penhale, 1993). The concept of elder abuse has most readily been accepted in countries of northern Europe and Scandinavia (Denmark, Germany, The Netherlands, Norway, Sweden, and the UK) (Eastman, 1984; Dieck, 1987; Stang, 1986; Pritchard, 1992), and there is a rapidly growing body of analysis in France (CLEIRPPA, 1990; Marin, 1992). In other countries the family appears to have for rather longer remained a social institution relatively immune from criticism, although there is evidence that this is changing for example in countries as socially diverse as Greece and Norway (Hydle, 1989; Stathopoulos and Amera, 1992). In addition, the denigration of older service users by professionals on the grounds that they place a 'burden' on services, or the actual harming of older service users by professionals does not appear to be characterised as abuse in most countries (Council of Europe, 1992).

The lack of agreement on an operational definition of what constitutes elder abuse has not impeded the beginnings of a policy and professional practice response in those countries where the concept is accepted. A UK report, for which social workers and other professionals produced case examples, stated that:

> Action to alleviate abuse cannot wait for its incidence to be established. There is much evidence of its prevalence. The large number of cases produced for this study was surprising both to [the Social Services Inspectorate] and to the staff of the participating [Social Services Departments]. (Social Services Inspectorate, 1992, p. 19)

It is proposed that the refining of the problem through research and debate should continue at the same time. From the German perspective, Dieck (1987, p. 3110) similarly advocates research to gather more detailed evidence for precisely what is happening at the same time as families are offered active support (that is, intervention), describing the philosophy as one of help before the labelling of actions. In both cases the basis for this policy preference (simultaneous action and research) is based on the ethical position that as it is known that some people in situations of relative power-lessness are being harmed there is a moral obligation on professionals to respond, and that the interests of older people are not best served by stand-ing back in the guise of scientific methodology. Other methodologies, such as the use of discussion groups of self-identified abusers or other qualitat-ive techniques as both therapeutic and research tools may enable the prob-lem to be more clearly defined while at the same time offering immediate help to both victim and perpetrator.

The social location of elder abuse is difficult to determine. Structural issues, such as gender, race and class are sometimes absent from work on this topic, and many of the studies that have been undertaken do not allow methodologically for wide generalisation on these points. For example, in two recent examples of small-scale research there was a small gender imbalance, in that abusers appear to be slightly more likely to be men than women (although not to any great extent). In other studies the proportion of men is greater but it is still not statistically significant (Stang, 1986; Kurrle *et al.*, 1991; Social Services Inspectorate, 1992). However, given the greater proportion of women than men caring for older people this may indicate a greater tendency for men to abuse, a finding which is consistent with other observations of domestic violence (Dobash and Dobash, 1992). The higher number of women being abused can be explained also by the gender ratios of old age (Steinmetz, 1988; Council of Europe, 1992). In this sense elder abuse could be said to be an issue for women, although gender (of abuser or elder) is only one dimension identified in the pathway analy-sis presented by Steinmetz (1988).

Race and class are frequently absent from discussions of these issues, with some exceptions. The conclusion reached by Steinmetz (in the USA) that there was no statistically significant difference between black and white families in the incidence of abuse suggests that the Social Services Inspectorate report is correct to assume that any lack of comparable evidence in the UK stems from a continuing inaccessibility of services to black and other ethnic minority people (Steinmetz, 1988, p. 81; Pritchard, 1992, p. 11; Social Services Inspectorate, 1992, p. 20). Any issues of class remain to be inferred, because although it may be expected that poverty or low income and associated housing problems would be major stressors, they are only part of a range of possibilities and there is no statistical relationship with the outcome of abuse (Dieck, 1987, p. 312; Steinmetz, 1988). In other words, abuse of older people by caregivers may happen in many different contexts, in which psychological as well as social factors will play a part.

Resources for response are a matter of having both an identified policy and professionals who are trained and supported to undertake this role. Here again the variance between North America and Europe is important as the resources in many states of the USA include a 'requirement to notify' on the part of all professionals who come into contact with older people in the course of their work (Blakely and Dolon, 1991). Notwithstanding the estimate quoted by Blakely and Dolon (p. 184) that five out of six incidents are not reported, this does create a very different basis from the situation pertaining in Europe (Dieck, 1987; Council of Europe, 1992; Social Services Inspectorate, 1992). Indeed, it is on this point specifically that Dieck (1987, p. 308) bases her critique of the transfer of North American approaches to understanding and intervening in incidents of abuse, to Germany and other European contexts. It affects both the procedural basis for intervention and the professional construction of events, as it may be more important to offer assistance to an elderly person and a family carer separately from determining whether or not abuse has occurred. Such an approach will affect the type of help given and so is likely to be contentious between professionals and in wider society.

The other major resource for response is seen to be a body of appropriately trained professionals who are able not only to identify abuse and neglect but also to be able to place incidents within an understanding of the needs of older people and the impact of these on carers (Pritchard, 1992). A lack of such trained professionals is noted in the UK report (Social Services Inspectorate, 1992, p. 20), and this is echoed for all European countries (Council of Europe, 1992). However, the study undertaken by Blakely and Dolon (1991) in the USA suggests that it is not only basic skills, knowledge or values which are important in how professionals respond, but also the context in which they are employed. The occupational groups which were perceived as most helpful in responding to situations of elder abuse were nursing and social service staff who were community- (rather than hospital-) based, and none of the occupations was considered to be very helpful in the treatment of abuse or neglect. As Blakely and Dolon recognise, (1991, p. 194) 'relative access to victims and the types of service which can be provided' are key factors. This leads other agencies and the public to bypass sources of help because of the way in which

agency policies and priorities are perceived, and for agency-employed professionals to respond to those aspects of a situation for which they have
resources. (This finding matches more general conclusions about the
impact of agencies on professional practice in the UK and elsewhere; for
example, see Sainsbury *et al.*, 1982; Hugman, 1987). As a consequence,
the recognition by European agencies that policies and resources are an
essential aspect of identifying and intervening in instances of elder abuse
appears wholly appropriate (Vierter Familienbericht, 1986; Dieck, 1987;
Hydle, 1989; Pritchard, 1992; Social Services Inspectorate, 1992).

Another possible response has been to argue that, as the abuse or neglect
of older people is part of the range of adult human relationships they
should not always be dealt with separately, but sometimes as aspects of
wider family violence and distress (Callahan, 1988; Phillipson and Biggs,
1992; Pritchard, 1992). Indeed, this is the response made in some instances
in Australia, Canada and the USA (Leroux and Petrunik, 1990; Kurrle *et
al.*, 1991). Instead of seeing the phenomenon as 'abuse' this response may
refocus attention on to acts defined in legal terms, such as intimidation,
theft, assault and rape. Criminal and civil laws exist in all European countries to which older people potentially have recourse and so in theory it
would be feasible for all situations in which older people are harmed to
take action through the police or a lawyer (Council of Europe, 1992). In
addition, where people are prevented from acting for themselves because
of mental incapacity in some countries there is protective legislation which
can be used (Eastman, 1984; Dieck, 1987; Hydle, 1989). However, as with
other instances of family violence, there is a reluctance on the part of older
people to use legal means to deal with abuse (Breckman and Adelman,
1988). Not only is the person perpetrating the abusive acts very likely to be
a close relative but in addition that person is most probably the main or sole
carer. This may discourage older people or other relatives from seeking
help, either because of their feelings for the 'abuser' or because they
cannot envisage alternative sources of care (Homer and Gilleard, 1990).

It is possible also that the response of health and welfare agencies may
be discouraging if their main resource is in residential care and involves the
elderly victim being removed from the situation (Wolf and Pillemer, 1989).
In most contexts this is the last resort, and other community-based inter-
ventions are offered, including counselling (for both abuser and victim),
home-care support, and assistance with practical problems such as housing
or finance (Eastman, 1984). This is not the same as simply offering services
which do not have a direct bearing on the perceived abuse, which has been
shown to be ineffective (see Homer and Gilleard, 1990). In situations
where residential care for the older person is the sole available response, it

has been argued by the British Gerontological Society that an admission to care should only be with the explicit agreement of that person, the same perspective as that which pertains in the USA, where self-determination of the older person is a core value (Social Services Inspectorate, 1992). For this reason it appears to be important that, although a transfer of ideas from the field of child abuse may be useful, a too ready adaptation of child abuse procedures is not followed and in that sense this type of domestic violence should be regarded as being distinct (Dieck, 1987; Penhale, 1993).

In some senses, the issue of neglect (and also some aspects of 'psychological abuse') is a more difficult arena than demonstrable physical abuse in which to construct policy and professional responses. The very concept of neglect is based on moral rather than legal precepts, containing elements of social obligation and normative expectations about what ought to happen within care giving relationships (Finch, 1989; Pitkeathley, 1989). This is not the same as distinguishing between different types of causation (such as 'caregiver stress' versus 'malevolent motive' (see Breckman and Adelman, 1988, pp. 59–64) but the recognision that definitions of the neglect of needs or obligations must depend on the prior social delineation of those needs and obligations. This is not to deny that in some instances carers neglect or actually harm older people, but to identify that stress may arise from the contradiction between expectations and available resources (financial, emotional or practical), or because carers do not share the general view of social norms.

The normative perspective on abuse and neglect provides a possible indication for the relative lack of recognition in southern and eastern Europe. As was discussed above, in these countries there is a stronger 'family ideology' about caring when compared to northern Europe and Scandinavia (Lisón-Tolosana, 1976; Nazareth, 1976; Dontas, 1987; Midre and Synak, 1989; Sant Cassia, 1992; Stathopoulos and Amera, 1992). There are three possible explanations for the relative 'non-appearance of elder abuse' in the south and east:

1. That the strong ideology of family care serves as a limitation on both the perpetration of family violence and the neglect of perceived needs and obligations;
2. That the strong ideology of family care serves as a limitation on the extent to which it is feasible to discuss publicly the possibility of 'elder abuse'; and
3. That the strong ideology of family care serves as a limitation on the extent to which professionals intervene in families and have the opportunity to 'discover abuse'.

In the absence of further evidence these possibilities must remain hypothetical. Inferences drawn in Germany, Scandinavia or the UK from the USA and Canada have been shown to be relevant to some degree but also to have distinct limitations. Similar cultural and structural differences between different parts of Europe suggest caution should be exercised in the transfer of ideas (Dieck, 1987; Penhale, 1993). Even if older people are harmed or neglected (in professional as well as family contexts) the sense of 'shame' that is prevalent in countries such as Greece, Portugal or Spain may not only act as a barrier to the disclosure of abuse but also to structure possible responses. Those countries in which the idea of 'elder abuse' has been most readily accepted are those that have the greater use of the welfare state as a supplement or substitute for the family in the provision of care to older people. That is, it is more widely acknowledged that some individuals or families may (at the many least) require assistance and support to accomplish the caring role and at the same time there are more available alternatives to an unsatisfactory situation, including both community based and institutional provision. Even in these contexts, however, there may be a reluctance to disclose abuse or neglect because of feelings of family loyalty and affection, as well as fear and uncertainty (Eastman, 1984; Dieck, 1987). This suggests that there is a connection between the personal and public opportunities for 'elder abuse' to be identified as such. As and when these criteria are fulfilled in other parts of Europe its prevalence may be found to be more widespread.

Respect and Abuse in Old Age: A Contradiction

Defining the contradiction

In this chapter I have focused particularly on the negative aspects of ageing and old age, in ageism and elder abuse. This runs counter to the observation by Victor (1987) or by Fennell *et al.* (1988) that old age can be regarded as a period of opportunity for many people, as opposed to a time of misery. Living standards for many older people in Europe have risen in recent decades, and the poverty which I discussed above is not experienced by all older people (Pitaud *et al.*, 1991). Fennell *et al.* (1988, pp. 15–17) do go on to identify the social cleavages which characterise older people as a part of society: that it is more accurate to write of different groups of older people. However, it is important not to overstate the boundaries between such groups. In relation to each aspect of the lives of older people, whether it be income, housing, race and ethnicity, gender or family relationships, the range of circumstances and experience form a continuum as opposed falling into discrete categories. Moreover, these aspects of life overlap: one may be in poverty yet have supportive family relationships (or not), how this is experienced may relate to gender, or racial and cultural background (or both), and so on. Just as this may produce a variety of individual experiences of old age, so the ways in which different older people perceive their status as being valued or devalued will vary according to expectation and opportunity. Respect and abuse may be felt by degree as well as be observable in distinct categories.

Aspects of some negative attributes of ageing, notably ageism, appear to be universal. A person can be dismissed as 'a wrinkly' or 'a crumbly' subtly as well as blatantly in a variety of contexts, and as we saw earlier, to be called 'grannie' in Greece may be negative as well as positive depending on context. Even the older members of royal families (in those European countries which still possess this phenomenon) may be held to be 'good for their age' in a way which is patronising, irrespective of the extent to which they retain power and comfort through wealth and social position. The middle-aged redundant executive may face exclusion from the employment market because firms want to recruit people aged under 45 (or 40, or 35). Both these examples have a common cause with the elderly former manual worker dependent on a state pension, in so far as all three situations are defined in significant ways because of their chronological age (although I do not intend to minimise the differences, as emphasised by Victor, 1987, p. 2, pp. 24–5).

Negative values of ageing and older people have been stressed because this reflects the general tone of concern within social gerontology across Europe. In many countries over several decades there has been a consideration by some academics, professionals and policy makers of the ways in which older people have been ignored or actively discriminated against on the grounds of their age. The critical strand of thought in social gerontology has sought to make clear the reality of life faced by many older people against a more widespread belief that European societies are 'caring' or 'just'. The work of Rosenmayr (1969) in Austria, de Beauvoir (1977) in France, and Townsend and Wedderburn (1965) in the UK are among the more widely known early examples. In the decades since then the identifiable social ambivalence towards old age has not lessened, despite the improvements in living standards which were noted above (Featherstone and Hepworth, 1990; Pitaud *et al.*, 1991).

This observation brings the discussion back to the way in which the contradiction between respect for and abuse of older people is interwoven with the distinction between old age in general as a low-status part of the life-cycle, and older people as valued individuals, whether generally as fellow citizens or personally as people we know. It is as if the 'elderly people' who constitute a 'burden' in a 'demographic crisis' are not ourselves, our family or our friends. Old age is political precisely because it involves the struggle over definitions about our society and the place we and others occupy within it, and the value we attach to roles and relationships (Phillipson, 1982; Walker, 1986b). The continuing evidence is that in European society there is deep ambivalence and that old age remains highly contested territory within which the attributes of respect and abuse form a contradiction.

Towards a 'new' old age?

The impact of social gerontology on debates about the status and value of old age and older people is not clear-cut. This is not surprising, because it is a multidisciplinary field as well as drawing on differing value positions. Nevertheless I want to identify two specific approaches within the field to the question of social responses to older people, each of which has a contribution to make to the possibility of rethinking old age. These are:

1. The focus on whether or not society offers appropriate and sufficient help to those older people who have dependency needs – the 'caring' society; and
2. The focus on whether older people are accorded equal rights with other citizens irrespective of their age – the 'just' society.

The concern about care for older people comes from the 'remarkable documentation on the failure of the professions and the services to respond to the health, environmental and psycho-social needs of the aging' (Amann, 1980b, p. 191). As Amann notes, this does not mean that anything which can be labelled as a 'need' should or could be satisfied, or that it makes assumptions about whether such a response should be made by the state, by private action or a combination of the two. What it does point to is the necessity for social gerontology to be concerned about questions of the definition of needs and the responses made to them. Similarly, various comparative studies have focused on the issue of care in relation to ageing (Little, 1979; Palmore, 1980; Hunter, 1986; Jamieson, 1990; Kraan *et al.*, 1991).

There is an implicit connection in this approach that those older people who experience the greatest discrimination are those who, because of the effects of old age or the social construction of their lives as older people, have specific needs: for financial assistance, for mobility, for health care or for help with daily living tasks. So it is this group of older people about whom concern is principally expressed, and wider interest in ageing and older people forms a background to this end.

In contrast, the concern with rights is based on the premise that although there is a high incidence of need among older people (with levels of physical disability increasing with age) the focus on issues of welfare can pathologise old age and ignore the extent to which needs arise because of poverty, poor housing, lack of access to health care and so on (Johnson, 1976). The priority claimed by Fennell *et al.*, which was identified in Chapter 1, is 'to demonstrate both the "normality" and the diversity of older people and to encourage more wide-ranging perspectives than [those which] have dominated the field' (Fennell *et al.* 1988, p. 177). Their suggestions that social gerontology should look at elderly nudists, or focus on groups of older people from northern Europe taking extended winter holidays in warm climates is not to ignore very real problems faced by others, but through a consideration of the range of experiences in old age to understand the normal diversity. The concern with levels of pension or care are thus placed in the context of questions of why and how some people are discriminated against and excluded from aspects of life, while others are not.

The implicit connection in this approach is between the question of basic rights afforded to any person as a citizen of an advanced industrial country, as regards income, housing, food and participation in social life and the divisions between different groups of older people. Interest in who goes to the Canary Islands for the winter and who has to remain in a poorly-heated flat in Amiens, Copenhagen, Hamburg, Oslo or Sheffield (or Madrid, Milan or Thessaloniki) has a basis in the demarcation of those situations in which old age may be problematic from the many instances in which it is enjoyable and problem-free.

Both these approaches may partly claim a link with the social science of the 'underside' advocated by Townsend (1958) and Becker (1967) or the connection between social science and social problems suggested by Rein (1976). However, they differ from each other in their perspectives and in the extent to which particular writers are critical of social structures. Are they, then, in conflict, or is there common ground? Certainly, both can be said to lead to the posing of some fundamental questions about the quality of life for many older people in Europe: the former by establishing the range of needs and then examining the scale of provision; and the latter by exploring the breadth of normal life in old age and distinguishing differential access and discrimination. Where they contrast is in the emphasis they place on how ageing might be understood (the extent to which it is associated with need), whether older people who are wealthy and powerful are the proper concern of social gerontology in the face of high levels of need among some groups, and the continuing marginalisation of older people in many areas of life. So although it is pertinent to try to avoid the pathologising of old age (Johnson, 1976), it is necessary to consider the forms of care and other responses to need in old age, especially as this constitutes the major social response to ageing. It is with this is mind that I will in the next two chapters address patterns of welfare provision for older people.

These two approaches might also have common ground in that they are in principle opposed to the recent phenomenon of an explicit 'age war' in which US politicians and campaign groups, even gerontologists, have argued that older people 'have a duty' to 'disappear' or reduce their expectations of living standards to 'make room' for 'our children' (de Jouvenal, 1988, p. 47; Johnson and Falkingham, 1992). There are clear echoes here of the social attitudes from other times and places noted in this and earlier chapters, only now it is standards of living rather than actual physical survival which is at issue (Guillemard, 1983; Pitaud et al., 1991). This contrasts with the more widely claimed European view that older people are a group entitled to support from the welfare system (Victor, 1985), but in the context of ambivalent or contradictory values such support cannot simply be assumed, and it is possible that this may become an even more contentious issue in the near future. In such a situation the rights of people who have health and social needs are likely to be challenged even more in a process which could further devalue many older Europeans.

5

Older People and the Welfare Response

Types of Welfare

A range of services

Because older people may so often be typified either as 'retired' or as 'dependent', or both, there is a concentration of social responses to ageing, in public policy and professional practice, towards the meeting of needs. Such responses take the form either of financial and practical support, or of social and health care. An important characteristic of Europe as an advanced industrial society is the range of provision for older people (Little, 1979; Jamieson, 1991a). Cross-national reviews demonstrate the similarities of types of response in the different countries, although they also reveal wide variations in the extent to which any one service may be available (Little, 1979; Amann, 1980b; Hunter, 1986; Jamieson, 1991a). While a degree of generalisation is possible, it is important also to consider cross-national differences. In this chapter I will begin to examine the range of services for older people which have developed in European countries, emphasising the interconnection between the dimensions of such services concerning questions of where older people live and any care which they may receive. The discussion is focused on a typological approach to understanding the varying pattern of services in Europe. The chapter concludes by examining questions about who uses and who benefits from these services.

Financial and material support

Pensions as the predominant form of financial assistance for older people have already been discussed, particularly in Chapter 3. Retirement pensions exist in some form in all European countries. In addition to this basic support, there is a variety of financial and practical assistance available to older people in the form either of subsidies and discounts, or specialised provision, notably in relation to transport and to housing (Bornat *et al.*, 1985; Fogarty, 1986; Pijl, 1992; Széman, 1992). Although the levels of provision are much higher in north and west Europe compared to the south and east, the broad types of service offered are similar. For example, assistance with transport in the form of subsidised fares on trains and buses has been widespread across Europe for some time, although this is very limited in Greece and Spain, and regional in Germany (Palmore, 1980; Leeson *et al.*, 1993). In a few countries (especially France, Germany, The Netherlands and the UK) there are also special schemes using adapted vehicles and flexible schedules to improve access for people with disabilities, of which many users are older people. Belgium and Denmark also have a number of such schemes, but these are much less common (Tinker, 1981; Fogarty, 1986; Daunt, 1992).

Various types of leisure activity are offered at a discount to older people in most countries, ranging from attendance at cultural or sports events to foreign travel. These are usually made available either on the basis of an individual being in receipt of a retirement pension or of being over a specified age, with no other criterion of eligibility (such as level of income) (Blommerstijn, 1980; Huet and Fontaine, 1980; Bornat *et al.*, 1985; Kraan *et al.*, 1991; Leeson *et al.*, 1993).

These financial subsidies and supports are widely reported to be popular and well-used by older people. Indeed, subsidised transport may be essential for the use of other services or for the maintenance of social networks, a need which can be quite marked in rural areas (and which can be obscured to policy-makers) (Wenger, 1984 and 1988). However, there is a question about the basis on which support should be provided. Is age as a criterion in itself discriminatory, as in the entitlement of all people aged over 55, 60 or 65 years irrespective of their circumstances, or should these benefits be restricted to grounds of income, disability, and so on? This is a complex sociopolitical dilemma, and the diversity of arrangements in different countries points to a general reluctance to produce clear policies (Bornat *et al.*, 1985; Daunt, 1992; Leeson *et al.*, 1993). In practice, it is easier for welfare benefits, for which professionals or officials act as gatekeepers, to be based on judgements about 'need' while those offered by private commercial organisations are likely to use general criteria (such as possession of a pension book or identity card showing date of birth) and so include all people over a certain chronological age.

Financial and other support provided for older people's housing needs tend to be more readily rationed precisely because they are provided through professionals and officials. Where the benefit is in the form of direct payment this can be assessed against an individual's other income, being provided for those who are deemed to have insufficient income from other sources and taking the form of a supplement to pensions (Friis, 1979; Florea, 1980; Kraan *et al.*, 1991). The other main form of housing assistance is the actual provision of housing specifically designated for older people (de Beauvoir, 1977; Lowy, 1979; Hunter, 1986; Fennell *et al.*, 1988; Rose, 1993). Of the EC and Scandinavian countries only Belgium, the Irish Republic and Greece either do not appear to have or have only recently begun to develop such provision (Hunter, 1986; Teperoglou, *et.al.* 1990; Carroll, 1991; Stathopoulos and Amera, 1992). In Eastern Europe.too this type of housing either is not available or is a recent innovation (Hrynkiewicz *et al.*, 1991; Széman, 1992; Rose, 1993).

Some Western European examples of supported housing include flats or apartments which are let only to older people, while others – 'sheltered housing' or 'service flats' – constitute a degree of care in the form of a 'warden' who is available to give small amounts of direct assistance and to provide surveillance ('checking up to see if the older person is allright'), or shared social areas, or both. Such accommodation is often popular, especially where the alternative might be residential care, but is not without problems (to which I will return later) (Middleton, 1987; Fennell *et al.*, 1988; Bianchi, 1991). The presence or absence of a warden may be said to constitute a boundary between housing *per se* and forms of direct support, between the definition of services on grounds of residence and of care. As will be evident in the following discussion, this distinction is useful in considering the contribution made to the lives of older people by specific forms of social intervention. Technological developments, such as alarm systems, intercoms and the use of radio-telephone and computer links, are making this an increasingly flexible form of service which is minimally intrusive in the day-to-day life of the older person (Tinker, 1981; Allen *et al.*, 1992). It should be noted, however, that the cost combined with the attitudes of many older people make these patchy and as yet limited developments, more evident in the north and west of Europe than in other places (Kraan *et al.*, 1991).

Domiciliary services

A type of provision which does not require the older person to move to it. as it is based on the home of the older person, is domiciliary care. This type of care has been available in some form and to some extent in most of the EC and Scandinavian countries and in parts of Eastern Europe for many years (Little, 1979; Smolic-Krkovic, 1979; Florea, 1979 and 1980; Amann,

1980a; Fogarty, 1986; Hunter, 1986; Midre and Synak, 1989; Jamieson, 1991a; Daatland, 1992). In some countries of south and east Europe, notably Greece, Hungary, Poland, Portugal and Spain it is a more recent innovation (Hrynkiewicz *et al.*, 1991; Anderson, 1992; Stathopoulos and Amera, 1992).

Domiciliary care may be said to be an approach rather than a specific service, in that the term covers both social and health care, including domestic work, meals-on-wheels, personal care, home nursing and reme- dial therapy (Jamieson, 1991a). I have excluded domiciliary consultations with general medical practitioners, social workers and so on, although these may be part of the process leading to the provision of care services. Not all of these services are available in all contries, however and there may also be differences between urban and rural areas (Carroll, 1991; Henrard, 1991). What characterises domiciliary provision is that it consti- tutes care (sometimes at quite high levels) in which any residential compo- nent is based on the person's own home or the ordinary home of a family or substitute carer (including sheltered housing or serviced flats), rather than requiring a move into a communal context.

Day care

There is another group of services, neither integrated with residence nor provided to an individuals own home, which collectively may be termed 'day care'. The most common form of this is the social centre, which appears in some guise in all European states. Hospital care (distinguished from 'out-patient' consultations) is also available on a day basis in some countries (for example Denmark, France, Italy and the UK), often orientated towards rehabilitation (Brocklehurst, 1978; Friis, 1979; Hunter, 1986; Collins, 1989), although older people in most countries make use of hospitals as mainly in-patients (Jamieson, 1991b). In Greece in recent years a composite of health and social care centres have developed, the 'Open Care Centres for Elderly People' (KAPI), although the health com- ponent resembles the out-patient consultation pattern of the 'poly-clinics' (a form of multidisciplinary out-patient service) in other countries rather than the day hospital as such (Teperoglou, 1980; Teperoglou *et al.*, 1990; Blommerstijn, 1980; Collins, 1989; Minev *et al.*, 1990). The KAPI will be discussed in more detail in Chapter 7.

Respite and short-term residential care

Residential care – that which requires the older person to reside somewhere other than their own home to receive it – forms a qualitatively different pattern of care. One type of residential care provides 'acute' or short-term help in crises, to enable rehabilitation or to provide respite for informal carers (Holstein *et al.*, 1991). Again, this includes both social and health services, either of which may be utilised for a short-term period, in a planned way or in an emergency. The social services used in this way are almost universally designated for older people, while the health services are most likely to be demarcated by medical specialisation (cardio-thoracic, orthopaedic and so on), or for rehabilitation (Willcocks, 1983; Hunter, 1986). In so far as medical specialisation does not include geriatrics, the question of age should perhaps be of little relevance. However, there are instances where both individual and institutional ageism may have an impact, and chronological age may be used as a judgement in the allocation of a service. The common feature of this type of service is that the older person returns to his or her own home in the same way as any member of any other age group. However, as a distinct service type it is not prevalent (see, for example, Evers and Olk, 1991).

An example of an innovation intended to bring together the benefits of residential care while avoiding the problems of institutional life has been that of 'family placements' or 'boarding schemes', in which the older person lives in the home of a non-related paid carer, usually for a short period (although it may be long-term). More recently this model has been adapted to provide up to 24 hours care per day in the older person's own home to substitute for an absent family carer. This type of response can be seen as bridging domiciliary and residential care; it is one that, despite being based on 'paid volunteers' can provide care at an intensive level. There is no obvious pattern to the development of this approach, which can be seen in France, Hungary, the UK and parts of the former Yugoslavia (Marshall and Sommerville, 1983; Servian *et al.*, 1990; Welch and Boyd, 1990; Hrynkiewicz *et al.*, 1991; Rusica *et al.*, 1991; CLEIRPPA, 1992).

Long-term residential care

Finally, there are the types of provision which can be termed long-term or 'chronic' care. Long-stay hospital facilities, nursing homes and social care homes are the three major types, of which examples can be seen in differing combinations in all EC and Scandinavian countries (Hunter, 1986; Henrard, 1991; Daatland, 1992). The common features of these services are a relatively high level of direct care, the pre-dominant management of all aspects of daily life by professionals; and that the place of residential care becomes the older person's residence. It is this type of provision to which the epithet 'institution' is usually attached (Goffman, 1968; Willcocks *et al.*, 1987).

The range of services

From domiciliary care to hospital care the range of services can be viewed as two inter-related set of two continua structured around the elements of residence and care. On the residence dimension there is the distinction between the older person's own home (in which they may have lived for many years as a younger adult) at one extreme, and at the other extreme an institution where older people live communally and to which they move late in life solely because they need care. On the care dimension the opposite ends can be defined in terms of the extent to which the support takes the form of an occasional social visit, through direct assistance with specific daily living tasks, such as the provision of meals, to full nursing care.

At their most extreme these two dimensions 'overlap' so that residence and degree of care appear to be closely related. For example, older people who receive meals-on-wheels in their own homes once or twice a week when compared to those who reside in long-stay hospital wards are illustrative of opposite ends of both continua. Mid-range examples, however, may appear more complex in their variations. For instance, let us consider intensive domiciliary care in the older person's own home when compared with sheltered housing that does not include direct assistance: the former combines low levels of communality with a high level of care, while the latter can be typified as involving moderate communality combined with a low level of care. In other words, the degree of communality in living arrangements is not necessarily directly related to the extent of care provided, although in practice there are a number of connections. While there is not a causally determining link, a degree of coterminosity has developed (for historical reasons, which will be explored in Chapter 6) with the result that, in many situations, the level of care provided and the level of communality

TABLE 5.1   *Degrees of communality in residence and level of care, by service type*

Service type	Communal residence	Level of care
Domiciliary care	Low	Low, moderate or high
Day care	Low	Low or moderate
Sheltered or service housing	Moderate	Low or moderate
Social care home	High	Moderate or high
Nursing home	High	Moderate or high
Hospital	High	High

in residence increase together. Across Europe there has been in recent decades a tendency for residential care to become focused increasingly on the needs of the more dependent older people (Hrynkiewicz *et al.*, 1991; Kraan *et al.*,1991; Pijl, 1991). This relationship of residence to care is a major issue in contemporary professional and policy debates about the care of older people (a point to which I will return later). The care/residence relationship is represented in Table 5.1. To examine each of these dimensions in more depth I will look at them separately in order to identify the issues which are specific, before proceeding to examine further questions about their interconnection.

Somewhere to live?

An important aspect of the reasons why income and financial assistance in old age is a crucial issue is indicated by the relatively large number of older people resident in poor housing in many European countries, sometimes despite measures taken by the state to increase the supply of good quality housing (Lowy, 1979; Huet and Fontaine, 1980; Victor, 1987; Fennell *et al.*, 1988; Teperoglou *et al.*, 1990; Széman and Sik, 1991). Huet and Fontaine (1980, p. 130) commented that older people in France did not take up new housing reserved for them because they were emotionally attached to existing dwellings no matter how unsuitable such accommodation might be for their needs. Although Huet and Fontaine implied that such attachment was sentimental and therefore irrational, they noted also that high rents and the necessity of moving to a new district might also act as deterrents. A similar mix of attitudes and low incomes have been noted over a long period of time to have limited the use of purpose built-housing in the Irish Republic, Greece and Italy (Little, 1979; Florea, 1980; Power, 1980; Zarras, 1980; Fogarty, 1986; Bianchi, 1991, Stathopoulos and Amera, 1992). These observations highlight three important points about the issue of accommodation for older people:

1. Questions of housing and income are very closely related – poor quality housing is often associated with low income;
2. Psychological and social factors are important factors in the choices made by older people – these do not always appear to be considered by professionals and policy-makers; and
3. The extent to which accommodation is an issue for older people is related to the need for care – for example, increased levels of disability may lead to a need for appropriately designed housing.

Moreover, it is vital that these three points are seen to be connected. The concern of professionals and policy makers is usually with housing as a material service (the built environment) to meet practical needs (for example, for level access), and ignoring what Jenks and Newman (1978, p. 252) called 'the external realities', which include social and psychological factors. In other words, a concentration on older people as being physically frail has tended to obscure both the financial and personal implications of housing provision and the links between them (see Fogarty, 1986, p. 30). It also ignores the right of older to people to exercise choice and to take 'risks' in living in accommodation which other people might not choose (Norman, 1980).

One form of dedicated housing which is relatively popular with older people, as I have noted above, is serviced or sheltered accommodation. Both are types of purpose-built housing development in which the residents share a need for a certain degree of care. This is related usually to age and disability, although there are schemes (such as in Italy) where disability may be the sole criterion, with no reference to age (Florea, 1980; Bianchi, 1991). There are some differences between the two types, as serviced accommodation usually refers to the central provision of services to a complex, such as catering, laundry and communal rooms, while sheltered housing usually refers to a group of dwellings where there is a 'warden' to provide surveillance and to act as a facilitator for access to other services as they are needed (Phillipson and Strang, 1985; Browne, 1990). In some countries, such as France and Germany, serviced and sheltered elements may be combined as well as offered separately,but in others, such as Denmark, Italy and the UK, they tend to be structured separately (although this is beginning to change) (Hunter, 1986). In The Irish Republic both patterns exist, in different parts of the country (Browne, 1990).

Much of the literature about serviced and sheltered housing has a eulogistic tone, as this provision combines security and assistance with independence ('my own front door'). However, studies of these schemes in the UK have revealed some problems, with both a lack of clarity in the role of the 'warden' and limited availability being seen as problems in their development (Phillipson and Strang, 1985; Middleton, 1987). In addition, Victor (1987, p. 147. notes a double bind, in that to become eligible older people need to show that they are 'in need' and yet are at the same time able to live independently. Nevertheless, such accommodation provides flexibility, choice and a relatively high level of independence in what remains a communal context.

Residential homes (whether 'social' or 'nursing' care homes), considered as a service defined in terms of residence, are more ambiguous.

Although they are not usually seen only in terms of care, unlike long-stay hospital wards, the extent to which care overlaps with residence is a key feature, as is the high level of communality. These are very public places in which to live one's life (Willcocks *et al.*, 1987). The dominance of care over residence is such that these facilities are not considered to be part of the housing stock: in all European countries they are regarded as being part of health and social care provision in the way in which they are funded and administered (Anderson, 1992). For all these reasons, such services are not widely seen as the first choice of older people or their families *for residential purposes*. From Greece to Sweden and from Hungary to the Irish Republic research evidence shows that residential homes are the 'last resort' (Power, 1980; Kraan *et al.*, 1991; Széman and Sik, 1991; Stathopoulos and Amera, 1992). There are other reasons why such provision may be acceptable or even desirable associated with the range of care available, to which I will return in Chapter 6. Recent developments intended to improve social or health care homes have included this dimension, making homes more 'homely' by dividing them into small units of four to six people, but such innovations are not widespread (Willcocks *et al.*, 1987; Henrard, 1991).

So there are two central elements of designated residences for older people which affect both their acceptability to older people and their wider implications: the question of personal 'independence' and debates about a risk of creating a 'ghetto' of elderly people (Little, 1979; Fogarty, 1986). In Germany there was in the 1970s a particular effort to encourage the former and avoid the latter through the use of building regulations which limit the density of special housing and require it to be near facilities such as shops, transport and so on (Lowy, 1979, p. 217). Such an approach was intended to promote independence while discouraging segregation, although more than a decade later little further seems to have been achieved (Evers and Olk, 1991). Similarly in Denmark sheltered accommodation may be established in 'ordinary' apartments, and former institutional resources are being opened up to the community, if slowly (Friis, 1979; Rasmussen, 1991). In Italy the integration of older people with younger adults who have needs related to disability is a different approach, one which overcomes age discrimination, yet is still at risk of creating a ghetto (of people with disabilities); however, the Italian approach forms part of a continuum which also includes elements comparable to those in Germany and Denmark, such as the accessibility of locations and the opening of services to the wider community (Florea, 1979 and 1980; Bianchi, 1991). In other European countries,housing appears generally to be segregated.

For some older people the choice of living only with other members of their own age group is a positive one. It may reflect the desire to avoid the demands of living with other age groups (such as the 'noise' of children and young people), or it may be an expression of a wish to live in a community where old age is the central rather than a marginalising attribute. The clearest expression of this choice can be seen in 'retirement villages', mainly found in North America but which have also developed in various parts of Europe (Fogarty, 1986). As a form of residence, however, these are undoubtedly to be seen as private dwellings; although they bring together a concentration of people in the same age group, the form of housing tenure is directly comparable to any other part of the society in which they are located. So although perhaps not easily regarded as ordinary housing they fit into this continuum as part of the end defined as 'individual private residence' and cannot be seen as a form of communal living.

So, in the sense of being a place to live, the steps from ordinary housing, through sheltered accommodation to residential homes is not a smooth gradation in degrees of communality, but one in which a sharp break is evident between those which can be seen as 'one's own home' and those which cannot. Even in a country with a tradition of accepting state care, such as Sweden, there is a preference for staying 'at home' because of the way of life in residential care; one may not feel 'at home' in 'a home' as a consequence of the high level of communality (Sundstrøm, 1986). In countries where communality is more culturally normative, such as Greece and Portugal, there are other reasons for not valuing residential care, such as prevailing attitudes to family roles and obligations: I will return to these in Chapter 6. For most older people, therefore, there must be a good reason to give up one's own home, and that reason is usually the need for care (Allen *et al.*, 1992). Consequently, care needs, which form the other of the two continua defined here, are closely linked with questions about residence in old age.

Needing care

The meaning of 'care' in this context, although having some cross-national variations, is broadly the same throughout Europe. There is a pan-European division between social and health care, at least in so far as concerns the organisation and administration of services, which is evident also in other developed countries such as Australia, Canada and the USA (Anderson, 1992; Kosberg, 1992). 'Social' care may be said to refer to those forms of assistance which supplement or replicate the older person's own daily living capacities, while 'health' care is concerned with the treatment or alleviation of illness or infirmity. However, practical demarcation is difficult to achieve, as health needs may have social consequences and vice versa (Brearley, 1978). The line is usually drawn by the institutional arrangements which are made for the delivery of care services. In a comparative reading of data from nine EC countries (Hunter, 1986), it is clear that while in some countries there is a balance between health and social services, in other countries a health perspective predominates in defining the care needs of older people. Indeed, in countries such as Belgium, France and Germany current policies to extend community services and home-based care (*maintien-à-domicile*) by increasing both home nursing and social welfare services is intended, to a large extent, to reduce the demands on the institutional health services (Jamieson, 1991b).

There are two possible reasons for the variability of this boundary. First, the medicalisation of old age (along with many other aspects of life) may cause social definitions of need to be seen as subsidiary. This can be seen as the ideological predominance of health. Second, several occupations which provide the relevant services are themselves defined as 'health professions' although individuals involved in them address both types of need, especially nurses and remedial therapists (Hugman, 1991). This is the institutional predominance of health. The ideological and institutional aspects are mutually reinforcing. Moreover, both draw on the underlying power of the 'sick role' in industrial society as a means of avoiding stigma in a situation of dependency, compared to social need, which may carry implications of moral unworthiness (Parsons, 1952; Abrahamson, 1991; Hugman, 1991; Kraan *et al.*, 1991). Dependence arising from health problems is more acceptable than for social reasons.

An example of differences in the health definition of need can be seen in the variable development of geriatrics as a distinct medical speciality. Of the EC countries, by the mid-1980s only in Greece was it totally non-existent, and in Germany, The Netherlands, Portugal and Spain it is a recent innovation (Blommerstijn, 1980; Hunter, 1986; Dontas, 1987; Anderson, 1992). In Greece emphasis upon geriatrics as a speciality is often regarded as a problem by other medical specialists, who consider the large-scale use of their resources by older people to be inappropriate; in Germany and The Netherlands geriatrics has developed contrary to an expressed policy preference for non-segregation. (A comparable situation was seen earlier in Norway, where geriatrics was a recognised speciality, but by 1980 there had been few designated geriatric in- patient facilities developed; see Beverfelt, 1980). In these instances, as in all other European countries, the medical view of the distinctive needs arising from biological ageing is highly influential. The capacity of the human body to resist illness

is seen to decline with age (although there is wide variation between individuals, as at any age) and there is an increased likelihood of several problems occurring at the same time, with an interactive effect (Briggs, 1990).
The influence of the medical perspective may contribute to ageism in that a
too-easy association between old age and illness, disease and disability
may be suggested; at the same time it is empirically observable that older
people consume the larger proportion of health budgets compared with any
other age group, reflecting an age-related prevalence of health problems
(Victor, 1987; de Jouvenal, 1988; Briggs, 1990; Anderson, 1992).

While health care is a major aspect of welfare provision for older people
across Europe, the institutional form it takes varies considerably between
countries. At one extreme, long-stay hospital care is provided in all EC
countries except The Netherlands, where all long-stay care is in nursing
homes (Hunter, 1986; Pijl, 1991). The extent of such long-term health care
also varies, and is dependent on the availability of alternatives. For example, other services do not exist in the same quantity in the Irish Republic as
in The Netherlands, and nursing homes constitute a greater proportion of
the care provided in the former than in other EC countries (Carroll, 1991;
Henrard, 1991). The general trend in Europe, however, is for such care to
be linked whenever possible to general adult medical services, through the
attachment of geriatric units to general hospitals, or via home-based health
care services (Jamieson, 1991a).

As was noted earlier, of the EC countries, only Denmark, France, Italy
and the UK have day-hospital provision, as opposed to out-patient care
(Hunter, 1986). In countries which do have day-hospitals, the service is
described as offering rehabilitative care while reducing the need for in-
patient facilities (see Brocklehurst, 1978). In this way it is cost-effective
and helps to maintain older people in their own homes. In theory, this
arrangement is very flexible, as the individual can have as many or as few
days' attendance as necessary, although limited resources, including transport, mean that the ideal of meeting all needs may not be reached. In fact,
attendance is often severely rationed so that only a fraction of those judged
by professionals to need this service actually receive it (Brocklehurst,
1978; Hunter, 1986).

A health perspective also predominates in some residential care systems.
In the Irish Republic, for example, homes which provide care that is (by the
definitions given above) primarily social, are nevertheless staffed by nurses
(Fleetwood, 1980; Carroll, 1991). In France, many residential homes are
registered for nursing care alongside social provision, but in Germany,
Italy, Spain and the UK nursing and social care homes are quite distinct
(Lobo *et al.*, 1990; Henrard, 1991). Again, it must be emphasised that the

boundary between the two is not very clear and, as noted above, there is a Europe-wide tendency for social care facilities to cater for rapidly increasing levels of infirmity. In practice, questions about whether or not older people are given appropriate forms of care rest ultimately on whether the skills of staff meet their needs and whether the home is institutional in terms of the environment created and the way it is run. Any judgement about the desirability of either model should arise from the actual care provided rather than from essential differences in 'types' of need.

However, in those countries where residential homes are divided between health and social care there must be some device for making decisions about allocation of places, at least for the majority of people who are supported by state funding or private insurance payments. In the UK, for example, state funding for a nursing home place requires certification by a doctor that the older person has a health need. However, because this does not eliminate the possibility of residents in social care homes having high levels of physical disability or mental infirmity, in some areas the difference between the two is entirely a matter of administrative arrangement. As Victor (1987, p. 296) observes, apart from state sector funding the only criterion for admission is the ability to pay, and many older people move into residential care because they can see no viable alternative. Consequently, it is possible to find nursing homes with residents who do not strictly need nursing care. All European countries have some similar administrative device, involving professionals (often doctors or social workers, sometimes both) in assessments which are likely to have a financial component as well as addressing physical and social needs; in Germany and Spain this results in lower levels of dependency in social care facilities (Lobo *et al.*, 1990). I will return in Chapters 6 and 7 to the question of the likely impact on such arrangements of policies intended to set stronger limits on the use of public resources.

As with residential care, domiciliary services can be orientated towards either health or social care. As with residential care, some provision is unambiguously social care (such as meals-on-wheels, which is universal in the EC and Scandinavia, at least by country, if not by region) and some health care (such as the administration of physical treatments). Yet here also the boundary between the two can be vague and the source of problems. In an instance of high dependency, the question may be very important to professionals and administrators with limited resources, as it becomes a device for determining responsibility It may,of course, be of only theoretical interest to the older person involved, who simply needs a service to be provided by *somebody*. Bathing, helping someone get in or out of bed, dressed or undressed, fed and to the toilet may be categorised as

110 *Ageing and the Care of Older People in Europe*

social or health care depending on the qualifications of whichever service is available, as evidenced by data from nine EC countries (Hunter, 1986). In many instances the only person available may be professionally unqualified, such as a family member, and this is an issue which I will explore further in Chapter 6. This is illustrated by the differences between France, where home nursing includes help with hygiene and daily activities, the UK where the former is usually a 'health' need and the latter 'social', and Germany, where both are likely to be the responsibility of a homemaker or home-care workers from social welfare agencies.

Those services, which are unambiguously defined as social care in all European countries: meals-on-wheels and home help with domestic tasks, have developed to provide directly the basic daily living tasks of cooking and cleaning. As was noted earlier, these are almost universal throughout the EC and in Scandinavia as well as in some parts of Eastern Europe (Amann, 1980b; Hunter, 1986; Hokenstad and Johansson, 1990; Henrard, 1991; Daatland, 1992; Széman, 1992). The form of these services does not vary much between the different countries, as for the most part they are regarded as rectifying deficits arising from increased frailty. Of course, whether or not services are made available may depend on whether frailty is accepted as a social and professional responsibility or is related to family obligations, as will be discussed further below. Home help is domestic work, involving cleaning, laundry, shopping and preparing food, while meals-on-wheels is the delivery of ready-prepared food. Such provision enables older people to maintain a reasonably normal life with dignity and it is highly valued, although in some countries there is a history of home-help workers being regarded as 'chars' or 'domestic servants' (Amann, 1980b; Harbert and Dexter, 1983). Harbert and Dexter (1983, pp. 62–71) also referred to the way in which they observed home help to be developing into home care in some countries including Finland, Germany, Switzerland and the UK, both by the way in which other tasks such as personal care are being assumed (with a resulting move towards a nursing role) and the way in which such tasks are performed to enhance and support the capacities of the older person, rather than emphasising deficits.

This change in focus has come at a time of fiscal pressures on services, which may in the future result in the diminution of domestic work provision in favour of personal care tasks (Harbert and Dexter, 1983; Henrard, 1991; Jamieson, 1991b; Daatland, 1992). In this way the policy of targeting domiciliary services on grounds of need may result in the loss of basic support for many older people. The implications of this for possible alternatives will be pursued in the next chapter; here it is relevant to note that as this type of basic service forms one end of the care continuum its reduction will reduce the range of provision to those people with the lowest level of need. As part of the benefit of this type of care is claimed to be the maintenance of independence amongst older people, then without viable alternatives any diminution can only produce short-term gains for policy-makers and service managers.

Patterns of provision

A typological approach to understanding the range of service provision systems has been used by Little (1979) and by Hunter (1986) to sketch the institutional pattern of provision between different countries. Little (1979, p. 150) uses the distinction of degrees to which welfare services for older people are institutionalised in any given country. By the designation 'institutional' she does not mean 'closed residence' in the way this term has come to be used (after Goffman, 1968), but the extent to which welfare services are formalised socially through organisations, professions and the state. The resulting 'spectrum of care' is a single continuum, ranging from 'residual', through 'early institutional', and 'institutional' to 'maximum institutional', each category comprising five elements: family care; residential care; public funding; training programmes; and domiciliary services. However, despite the use of language, according to Little, (1979, p. 149) this spectrum does not represent an even path which has been or will be followed by all countries. Rather, it represents a means of distinguishing different types at a point in time. Furthermore, a subdivision of categories allows Little to distinguish between specific aspects of provision as they have developed in any one country.

Hunter (1986, p. 84) similarly portrays a spectrum, but unlike Little this has only two dimensions, degrees of public ownership or control and degrees of public funding. This places Denmark on the same point as Greece, Italy and the UK in relation to proportions of funding, but on a different point with respect to ownership/control, for example. However, there is a broad correlation between the two characteristics in the way they are presented, with a rough agreement overall between degrees of ownership/control and funding.

In order to compare Little's 'institutionality' with Hunter's degrees of public organisation, the two spectra are presented in diagrammatic form in Table 5.2 (including only the European countries from Little's spectrum). For comparability, I have used the criteria established in these two analyses to add the Irish Republic and Italy as 'middle institutional' and Belgium as 'maximum institutional' to Little's spectrum; and Sweden as 'high public

TABLE 5.2   *Two spectra of welfare provision compared*

Institutionality/ public organisation	Little (1979)	Hunter (1986)
'Early'/low	Greece	Eire, Belgium, Netherlands
Middle	Austria, (Irish Republic) Germany, (Italy), Netherlands	(Austria), Germany
'Maximum'/high	(Belgium), Denmark, Sweden, UK	Denmark, UK Greece, Italy, (Sweden)

organisation' and Austria as 'middle' to Hunter's categories. The additions are indicated in brackets. It is also essential not to ascribe a direct equivalence to the categories used; they are presented in this way to compare their use as a means of distinguishing the level and complexity of services for older people between European countries. In particular, this diagram illustrates the similarities and differences in the ordering of countries.

The observable variation derives in part from social changes occurring in these countries during the period between the two analyses, but it is also a reflection of the relative weight placed by Hunter on the formal definition of public service organisation, seen as state welfare provision, and an implicit bias towards health services. In contrast, Little's spectrum is one of both health and social provision considered more broadly, with both formal and informal aspects taken into account, including service specialisation, levels of professional training and types of organised non-governmental services.

This distinction is underlined by a consideration of the relative placing of Greece and Italy. By highlighting Greece and Italy as having a high degree of public welfare organisation, Hunter is recognising that both have a formal commitment to develop welfare state provision for older people, as well as for others, within the framework of creating national health services. However, the same data also show that in both countries the fiscal situation is not conducive to the realisation of these policies, so that in Greece, health care is in a 'state of flux' (Hunter 1986, p. 42), while in Italy the transition to a national health service, begun in 1978, is 'not yet complete and will take many years' (p. 54). That in neither case has the formal policy intention yet been accomplished in practice is reinforced by other analyses, and on a broader basis neither Greece nor Italy could be said to have welfare states of the same extent as those of Denmark, Sweden or the UK (Giori, 1983; Dontas, 1987; Dontas *et al.*, 1991; Bianchi, 1991). What Hunter is recognising is that these countries have a formal policy commitment to develop welfare-state responses to older people (including in both cases a national health service). This dimension is missing from Little's analysis, with the result that while Hunter appears to emphasise formal policy development quite heavily Little seems to neglect it and thus appears to typify a country such as Greece inappropriately.

The typological approach, as exemplified by both Little and Hunter, may be useful for relatively broad differentiation, as both approaches do have utility in making comparisons between different countries in relation to key specified features. However, there are limitations inherent in the choice of variables, with the consequence that allocation of specific countries to designated categories is fraught with difficulty, especially when considering detailed points of comparison.

To explore the comparative range of services for older people it is necessary to consider a model which distinguishes different aspects of services as delivered in addition to the way in which they are organised. Such a model would maintain a clear distinction between different dimensions and would not attempt to reduce them to one dichotomous variable. From the earlier discussion of services in relation to issues of residence and care three factors can be identified which may be used to typify differences in the development of welfare for older people. These are:

1. Location – where the service is provided;
2. Duration – over what time period it is provided; and
3. Formation – how it is structured and organised.

Concentration on one aspect (such as formation, as in Hunter, 1986) can obscure the others, which may point to a highly-developed range of welfare provision for older people.

The question of the *location* of services relates to the extent of community- or institution-based responses to the needs of older people. Is the service provided in a person's own home, or do people have to go somewhere else to use it? If they do have to go somewhere else to use it, does the location stigmatise and segregate or does it enable older people to be part of the wider community? Clearly there is a difference here between receiving care in a hospital which only serves older people and one which caters for all citizens, for example. At the same time, the meaning of any particular service may be similar across a range of contexts, so that the tasks expected of a home nurse in practice may not, for example, be very different from a hospital nurse. The significance of location of a service will therefore be in the related factors it has for older people, such as any impact on relationships with relatives, friends and so on.

Duration of service provision concerns timespan at the point of delivery, in two ways. First, there is the number of hours per day, days per week or weeks per year in which a particular form of welfare might be available. Meals-on-wheels may be allocated by a number of visits in a week, while home care is provided for a given number of hours per day, and respite care is available for one or two weeks every so many months. There will be many other variants between and within these examples. This sense of duration is a reflection both of the type of service and the level of need it addresses.

Second, there is the question of whether welfare provision is available in the short or long term, whether it is available quickly in a crisis or only after a lengthy period of waiting. (It may be necessary on this criterion to distinguish also between formal intention as defined in policy and the operational reality.)

The *formation* of welfare responses to older people, whether they are professional or informal, social or health, or a mixture of these, and whether they are funded by the state, through independent insurance schemes, paid for directly at the point of use or a 'mixed economy' is in itself a complex set of questions. At the policy level it is the formation of services, as public, private or a mix, which has come in recent years to dominate debates about care for older people (Evers and Svetlik, 1991; Huston, 1991; Kraan *et al.*, 1991). Within these debates, the location and duration of provision are also important factors for people providing and using services, as well as questions of who does what, who pays, and how the answers are to be determined. Formation is not only a question of general structure but also of the relationships between different groups of people, including older people themselves as well as professionals, informal carers and policy-makers, in that it has to be related to consideration of space (location) and time (duration) as they affect the construction of older people's lives.

Using these criteria, it is possible to distinguish patterns of provision more widely within a country and between countries. Not only services which already exist, but also any perceived gaps can be considered in relation to questions of location, duration and formation. It is for this reason that the linking of Greece, Italy and the UK as being of the same 'type' raises more problems for understanding the development of services than it solves. For example, although some aspects of their formation may be similar in that all are formally welfare states, the extent to which an insurance principle constitutes the basis of payment for services in Greece, part of that in Italy and only a small propotion in the UK mean that the reality of service type and availability will differ greatly for older people in each of these countries. There are considerable differences in the location of services, with very few domiciliary services in Greece, more in Italy and the greatest number in the UK. Again, service type understood by duration varies between these countries, with many more day services and short-term residential services in Italy and the UK than in Greece.

In this way it can be seen that types of welfare provision for older people are multidimensional and cannot easily be represented on a single spectrum. The current attempts to reshape welfare structures and practices across the EC, in Scandinavia and in Eastern Europe to which I have referred above revolve around just these questions, in terms of debates about institutional and community care. This will be examined in more detail in Chapter 6, and in terms of the wider relationship between ageing and welfare provision to which I will now turn.

Whose Services?

The social origins of old people's welfare

In order to consider the ways in which the services I have described have developed it is necessary to return briefly to the question of financial benefits. As I have outlined in previous chapters, the growth of retirement pensions, with all the implications this had for what it means to be old, was a major element in the development of the social creation of old age under capitalism (Phillipson, 1982). However, the provision of residential care in hospitals and other institutions goes back to medieval times, and even earlier. The almshouses and original hospitals of religious and civic charity (some of which survive) are the direct forebears of the old people's homes which are common across Europe (Amann, 1980b). Indeed, in the 'Mediterranean rim' countries (including France) this type of provision is still a part of the range of welfare responses to old age, despite being reduced in recent years. The ethos which prevailed in the charitable approach to welfare was one in which it was thought that assistance should be given only to those who lacked other means.

This brings the discussion back to the family, for although this cannot be assumed to be the *location* of all care for older people in all European countries (see Chapter 3) there is a widespread historical belief in all these societies that families do have some obligations towards meeting the needs of older people who require assistance. This sentiment is clearly expressed in the following observation by Charles Booth, a Victorian social reformer in Britain:

> To have lived at all goes for something, to have asked for no relief goes for more, and to have secured through savings, or through friendly feeling, or through the loving duty of children a chimney corner where 5s. a week will be adequate, may be accepted as proof that the pension is not ill bestowed (Booth, 1892, p. 237).

Dignified assistance for older people was 'earned' through the accumulation of one's own means or the obligations of friends and family. The first corollary was that socially valued welfare provision should be only for those who otherwise lacked sufficient means (that is, those who in some way could be defined as 'poor'). The second corollary was that they should be regarded as deserving of this assistance; for all others there should be only poor laws and handouts. Indeed, some professions concerned with helping older people, such as social work, emerged partly in response to the allocation of different provision to the 'deserving' and the 'undeserving' poor (Parry and Parry, 1979; Abrahamson, 1991; Pijl, 1991). Moreover, it can be argued that this approach of 'less eligibility' was not so much an attempt to make use of existing family relationships as to put pressure on families to avoid the stigma of their elderly relatives receiving poor relief and so create a sense of obligation (Anderson, 1977; Finch, 1989). This enabled policy makers to differentiate between those who had and those who did not have other support on which to call, irrespective of their 'natural' relationships.

It is from this historical background that it can be said that old people's welfare has emerged out of social concerns either to support families in the care of their older members or to substitute for those families which are unable or unwilling to do so. The cost for those without family, or without family able or willing to provide care, was that of accepting the physical and social consequences of pauperism. As de Beauvoir noted about French facilities in the 1960s, in her analysis of a ministry of public health report:

> In the past an institution was a place for gathering the infirm, the bedridden and the healthy aged together with the one idea of giving them some slight degree of shelter, often in shocking promiscuity and with the minimum of food; everyone knew the formula. Unhappily, this same formula is still being widely used (de Beauvoir, 1977, p. 285).

In this way, welfare responses to old age have been laden with the stigma of poverty and other forms of social disadvantage. In Chapter 6 I will examine the contribution this background has made to the development of community care policies.

Indeed, in more recent decades there has been a substantial, although perhaps precarious, shift towards a reconstruction of welfare, based on the idea that services are a right of citizenship (Taylor, 1989; Siim, 1990). Allocation may be made through assessment of need, but the basis of the receipt of services has increasingly become the social relationship between the older person and the state or an agency of the state (such as an insurance company). Eligibility for welfare in modern Europe is based on payment of taxes and insurance contributions rather than the accumulation of moral worth. For those who can afford to pay, however, there may be a better standard of service, and in some eastern European countries until recently this may have taken the form of a bribe rather than a formal payment (Hartl, 1991, p. 34). For this reason it might be expected that a much wider group of older people not only need but also *want* to use the services that are provided, although I will return below to the possibility that 'moral worth', including the willingness of families to participate in the provision of care, continues to play a part in welfare service use.

Who uses these services?

Not all older people make use of welfare services. This may appear to be an obvious point, but it requires elaboration. Some older people clearly do not need to make use of welfare provision, other than the very widespread receipt of retirement pensions. To take the example of physical disability, it was noted earlier (see page 79) that although despite this being a major cause of dependency in old age, only a minority of older people have serious disabilities, so most older people either do not need help or need only minimal levels of assistance. The services discussed above are provided for the minority of older people. Estimates in the Irish Republic, Sweden and the UK, for example, of the proportions of older people using organised forms of help tend to be around 25 per cent (although estimates vary slightly between countries) (Walton, 1982; Hokenstad and Johansson, 1990; Carroll, 1991). So who are the people who use the services?

First, it is widely recognised that dependency needs increase with advancing age, and older elderly people are most likely to have recourse to organised assistance. The definition of later old age as 75 years is used here, although in some analyses the age of 80 years is used (Coleman and Bond, 1990; Kraan *et al.*, 1991). The reasons for this are the increase in disability which tends to occur among older elderly people, as well as increasing social isolation (for example, from the death of spouses, friends and associates). So the first distinction is that service use tends to be by the oldest members of society, in particular those who have a disability. Among younger old people service use tends to be related much more closely to disability alone.

Second, in all European societies there are more women than men in the older age groups (Eurostat, 1991). Given the previous point about the relationship between age and disability, this in itself should suggest that there will be more women needing care than men. In addition, evidence from Denmark, France, Germany, The Netherlands, Sweden and the UK suggests women are more likely also to live in single person households. This means that in Northern Europe the probability increases that older women will have a need for care from outside the household (Chauviré, 1987; Victor, 1987; Kempen and Suurmeijer, 1991; Thorslund, 1991). However, there is evidence also, at least in some countries, that older men, or households in which a man is the main carer for an elderly person, make use of greater levels of service provision than do women in similar situations – and men are more likely than women to be admitted to residential care (Finch and Groves, 1982; Teperoglou *et al.*, 1990; Wærness, 1990). The use of services appears to be gendered. What is not clear is whether this phenomenon does not, in fact, exist or is simply not reported in other national studies, given the European- wide greater longevity of women.

Third, class divisions can be identified in service use, in relation to both the extent and type of specific facilities utilised. For example, research in the UK has shown that the national health services are used mainly by the middle classes (defined as non-manual workers) among all age groups, largely because of greater knowledge about access (Townsend and Davidson, 1982; Anderson, 1992). This is despite the greater prevalence of ill-health and disability among working-class groups (defined as manual workers and unemployed people) in the former communist as well as in capitalist countries (Bonanus and Calasanti, 1986; Victor, 1987; Minev *et al.*, 1990; Rusica *et al.*, 1991; Széman and Sik, 1991). A comparable phenomenon has been identified in the use of social services in other countries, such as the Open Care Centres for Elderly People (KAPI) in Greece or day care in The Netherlands (Teperoglou *et al.*, 1990; Amira, 1990; Nies *et al.*, 1991). The one aspect of which working class older people (men especially) tend to be more prevalent users is residential care in the state and charitable sectors (Rhein, 1987; Grundy, 1989; Foster, 1991). In this there is a sense of continuity with the arrangements made for paupers, out of which modern charitable and state provision developed, but the private residential homes utilised more by the middle classes in Northern and Western Europe are based on an entirely different premise. The key factor here is the extent to which the services have come to be redefined as a right of citizenship or the benefit of private wealth (Foster, 1991; Rusica *et al.*, 1991).

Fourth, where there are racial or ethnic minorities, the use of welfare services by older members tends to be limited with regard to the racial or ethnic majorities, even taking into account the smaller proportions of older people in many ethnic minority communities (Fennell *et al.*, 1988; Cameron *et al.*, 1989; Williams, 1990). This is to be seen not only in the situations of migrants from former colonies (as in France, The Netherlands and the UK) but also in relation to migrants between EC countries (such as older Irish people in the UK) and other more recent migrant groups, as well as ethnic and racial minorities that have been long established (such as some Jewish or black communities) (Blommerstijn, 1980; Torkington, 1983; Norman, 1985; de Jouvenal, 1989; *Social Europe*, 1991). The racism faced by these groups, whether institutional or personal, may take the form of inappropriate services (for example, lack of ability to communicate with service users, cultural insensitivity), lack of access (including information), and even on occasions direct exclusion because of decisions made by professionals (Rooney, 1987; Williams, 1990). This has produced a debate in the UK, for example, about whether it is more effective for ethnic minority groups to establish their own services or to seek a proper response from the mainstream provision. While some critics argue that the changes necessary on the part of ethnic and racial majorities will be too slow to be effective, and so seek separate services which can be organised by minority groups, others claim that this will enable majority groups to avoid having to address the issues (Phillips, 1982; Torkington, 1983; Rooney, 1987). Certainly, there has been a lack of recognition among professionals and policy-making groups, including gerontologists, of the problems faced by racial and ethnic minority older people in gaining access to and using welfare provision, although this is now beginning to change (and there have been some exceptions) (Bhalla and Blakemore, 1981; Donovan, 1986; Cameron *et al.*, 1989; Pijl, 1992). Nevertheless it is still the case that services are readily more available to members of ethnic and racial majorities.

On each of these dimensions there are issues of inequality and discrimination in the construction, allocation and rationing of welfare provision. Although it is true in a formal sense that service use in all European countries is based to a degree on concepts of citizenship rather than charitable principles or moral definition, access to services is not open equally to all citizens. Whether or not an older person knows about, chooses and is given a service will be a product of that person's age, disability, gender, class and racial or ethnic background.

Who benefits?

The primary beneficiaries of welfare provision are older people themselves although, as we have just seen such people are not a homogeneous group, and white middle-class men appear to gain more than others. However, it is possible to suggest that there are real gains for many older people in the widespread development of welfare services in European countries. Indeed, the demand for some services points to popularity among older people. However, it should be noted that this is most apparent when the services are less stigmatising: for example, in general there is less enthusiasm for residential care, as shown in many studies (Sundstrøm, 1986; Dontas, 1987; Foster, 1991; Széman and Sik, 1991). Yet, irrespective of their popularity, welfare services have developed to support and assist older people in maintaining physical and social functioning to the extent that it is now synonymous with the idea of an advanced industrial society and used as a measure of development (Gilleard *et al.*, 1985).

In addition to older people themselves, some welfare responses have benefited family and other informal carers, directly or indirectly (Marshall and Sommerville, 1983; Jani-Le Bris, 1992). Informal carers may be supported by domiciliary services, day-care and short-term residential services which either share the work of caring on a regular basis or for fixed periods. Where a carer wants to continue looking after an older person, supportive services are essential. However, it has also been pointed out that in several countries the extent of welfare provision to individuals may be reduced because of the presence of a carer, with the consequence that other aspects of the carer's life become disrupted by this one relationship (Finch, 1984; Wærness, 1990; Bianchi, 1991). For example, Finch (1984) refers to evidence that the older person may not be allocated a home help because a daughter lives nearby, even if the daughter has other commitments. When this happens the family carer may feel that she (or he) is contributing to more than benefiting from the welfare system.

To what extent could it be said that wider society is a beneficiary of the welfare provided for older people? Undoubtedly there is some gain, in the form of employment for professionals and care workers, and it could be argued that a minimal level of welfare prevents the situation of the growing numbers of older people from becoming too socially disruptive (Amann, 1980b; Hrynkiewicz *et al.*, 1991). Yet this answer is only part of the picture, as evidenced by the recent attacks on welfare based on financial and social costs identified mainly with the political New Right, which have had an impact across Europe as well as in North America, and which are partly driven by a concern about the costs of the health and welfare needs of older people (Estes, 1986; Zapf, 1986; Binney and Estes, 1988; Saltman, 1991; Thorslund, 1991; Daatland, 1992). In Eastern Europe one economic consequence of the rapid political changes is a growing crisis in the support of older people as the predominant recipients of welfare (Széman and Gáthy, 1993). If the potential demands for welfare are unlimited, then constant growth (or maintenance at a time of economic decline) will be contested, especially when the recipients are not unambiguously a highly valued social group, as was discussed in Chapter 4.

In each respect, therefore, there is as great a sense of competing as of complementary interests in the patterns of European welfare provision for older people. The triangular connections between the needs, wishes, rights and resources of older people, informal carers and wider society cannot be assumed to be harmonious. There is a complex 'social economy of care' operating, in which concepts of exchange and reciprocity may form part of the vocabulary but in which many participants do not feel the exchange is equal or that reciprocity is being met. So while some older people, some carers and some aspects of broader society may be said to benefit, there are others for whom the welfare provided to older people remains at best contradictory.

Old Age and the Welfare Response

The welfare image of ageing

Despite the pressures currently being experienced on the ways in which services for older people are structured, financed and operated, there is at the same time a continuing widespread belief in the desirability of social provision for elderly people who need assistance to cope with the ordinary demands of living (Fogarty, 1986; Jamieson, 1991a). Although it is the minority of older people who are using such services at any one time, and the overall increases in the proportions of older people are seen by some observers as constituting a crisis, it is perhaps easy for these services to continue to receive generalised support because this reinforces the idea of the good society, while at the same time drawing on the one-dimensional view of ageing as a process of increasing dependence (Victor, 1985; de Jouvenal, 1988). A sense of contradiction arises precisely because welfare responses to older people are constructed simultaneously around negative images (decrepitude and dependence – irrespective of empirical evidence) and a positive valuing of individual older people (Minois, 1989). This may produce a pathologising effect in the expression of social concern (Johnson, 1976), but at the same time it is necessary to have a reason for intervention in people's lives, such as poverty or infirmity. These provisions are not made for all older people, only for those older people who do not have other means of resolving problems of daily life. Such difficulties may be experienced by many more without the need to make use of 'services', precisely because they have other resources.

The restructuring of welfare currently taking place in Western European countries could be said, therefore, not to be driven by a wish to prevent older people having safeguards against poverty or infirmity, but a wish to make as many people as possible responsible for their own life situation. This may be achieved through the increased use of insurance arrangements, which exist already in some countries (Belgium, France, Germany, and The Netherlands for example) and are gradually being introduced in others (such as Scandinavia and the UK). As so many more people can now be expected to live longer lives, issues such as income maintenance and health care are the concern of the majority and not just a few. This could be construed as a destigmatising development: everyone will need pensions and the availability of health care (just in case), so thinking about this must be a normal part of everyone's planning for the future. Within this approach, social and health needs are defined as being everyone's experiences, therefore normal and not pathological. However, as Estes (1986), writing from the North American experience, has so clearly expressed it, to the extent that such a model now predominates it has *commodified* social security. That is, it turns not only welfare services but also the needs of older people into a commodity to be dealt with on the basis of market forces. This may be an advantage to those social groups who have resources, but it is a disadvantage to those who do not. It is precisely because these latter groups form minorities (of class, gender and race as well as of age) that they should be within the focus of a critical analysis. The multiple marginalities that are likely to be reinforced in the future contribute to the growth of an underclass which appears to be emerging within advanced capitalist societies (Robinson and Gregson, 1992).

The alternative perspective to a 'welfare approach' in considering old age is to regard it either as just one stage of the life-course (stressing its normality) or else to argue that it only exists to the extent that policymakers, professionals and academics create the phenomenon of 'old age' through their delineation of it as a 'problem' (Fennell *et al.*, 1988). However, as Fennell *et al.* demonstrate, although ageing is a normal part of human experience, the relationship between our social structures and this part of the life-course do make it problematic for some people (see the discussion in Chapter 4), and the receipt or otherwise of welfare assistance for the most part centres around the experience of problems.

For these reasons I have concentrated in this chapter on the broad models of welfare provision for older people that have developed in Europe. There is a prevailing circularity in that the welfare structures of Europe are now dominated by particular groups of older people (those who require assistance) and so public interest in older people is focused more intently on the issue of their social and health needs. Although the majority of older people do not have welfare needs beyond the range seen in other adult groups, the question of care for elderly people is a major issue for European society as we approach the end of the twentieth century. We may wish to resist the equation 'old means dependent' as ageist (which it is), but the ageing profile of European society presents a challenge specifically to policy makers and professionals, as well as to society more generally, which appears likely to flavour the debates about ageing for the foreseeable future (de Jouvenal, 1988).

A possible alternative?

Is it possible to construct more 'positive' models of provision? If the existing patterns of social response are defined in terms of decrepitude, dependence, illness and infirmity, how can a viable alternative be constructed? Such an alternative would require a critical awareness of the difficulties faced by older people with social and health needs (for an income, mobility and assistance in daily living for example), while at the same time encompassing and stressing the positive aspects of old age.

Clearly, to meet this requirement the emphasis of services would have to be on the enhancement of ordinary life rather than on perceptions of deficit. This is not to deny the reality of disability, poverty or other difficulties faced by some older people. What I am suggesting is that if our focus were more on the nature of, causes of and solutions to specific difficulties, then a more common response between problems faced in old age and the difficulties faced by younger adults could be developed. This indicates a basis not only for common cause between people of different ages, rather than an age segregation, but also a learning by policy-makers and professionals from the debates taking place in other areas of service provision. These include the importance of recognising the social politics of the caring services and a consideration of the transferability of concepts and

124 *Ageing and the Care of Older People in Europe*

practices developed in services for other groups of people but which are also applicable to older people, offering models based on the idea of empowerment, ordinary living and so on (Oliver, 1990; Bianchi, 1991; Ramon, 1991). I will discuss these models further in the following chapters.

In this review of the various forms of services for older people a particular current has been noted in Europe, namely a tendency for questions of care to be related to the place of residence of older people. In all European countries there are forms of institutional life, including social-care homes, nursing homes and (with the exception of The Netherlands) long-stay hospitals. I have noted also that in recent decades there has been a movement towards the development of community services (defined as those not provided in institutions). Having in this chapter examined the different forms of welfare response to old age, and set these in a broad context, in the next chapter I want to turn to a more detailed analysis of the division between institution and community and to explore the meaning this division has given to the shaping of old age in modern Europe.

6

Institution and Community

Home or Away?

Two types of care

For those older people in Europe who need personal care the range available is defined, in broad terms, by whether or not it can be provided at

TABLE 6.1   Approximate percentage of people aged over 65 years using institutional or home-care services, late 1980s (all figures rounded to nearest whole per cent)

Country	Percentage institutions	Percentage home-care
Austria	3	2
Belgium	5	5
Czechoslovakia	6	5
Denmark	6	25
Finland	5	16
France	5	8
Germany	4	3
Greece	1	1
Hungary	1	3
Irish Republic	7	3
Italy	2	2
Luxembourg	Not available	7
The Netherlands	10	12
Norway	6	19
Poland	1	1
Portugal	2	1
Spain	2	1
Sweden	9	18
United Kingdom	6	9

Sources: Evers and Svetlik (eds) (1991); Anderson (1992); Daatland (1992); Jani-Le Bris (1992); Kosberg (ed.) (1992); Széman (1992).

home. Despite widespread variations in the balance of the different elements in care systems, this may be said to be the dominant European concern in social welfare for older people (Jamieson, 1991a). In this chapter I want to focus on developments taking place within and around the divide between institutional and home-based care services. Each will be examined in turn before more general trends are explored.

The proportionate use of institutional and home-based care services by older people differs between the countries of Europe, sometimes quite markedly. Table 6.1 provides a comparison between nineteen countries, showing the percentages of people aged over 65 who used the two types of formal services in the latter part of the 1980s. The figures are derived from several sources and do not all relate to the same year. In some cases they have been calculated from data available in national studies. Therefore, they must be treated as approximate.

The relationship of institution and home-care

These figures suggest that, in terms of proportionate usage, countries may be seen to form several distinct groups. In relation to institutions, there are the countries with relatively high usage (7 per cent or more), which are the Irish Republic, The Netherlands and Sweden. Then there are those with middle level of usage (from 4 to 6 per cent), which are Belgium, Czechoslovakia (as it then was), Denmark, Finland, France, Germany, Norway and the UK. Third, there are the countries with low proportions of institution usage (3 per cent and less), which are Austria, Greece, Hungary, Italy, Poland, Portugal and Spain. In relation to institutions, therefore, there would appear to be an approximate divide between the north and west and the south and east of Europe.

The pattern of proportionate home-care usage is slightly different. Here there are some very high levels of formal service use, 16 per cent and over, which identify Denmark, Finland, Norway and Sweden as countries with relatively widespread home-care usage. The middle levels, between 5 and 12 per cent, are to be found in Belgium, Czechoslovakia, France, Luxembourg, The Netherlands and the UK. Then there are the countries with low proportions of home-care usage, of 4 per cent and below, namely Austria, the Irish Republic, Germany, Greece, Hungary, Italy, Poland, Portugal and Spain. This latter group is notable, also, because with the exception of Hungary, home-care coverage is at a level equal to or below that of institutions.

Coverage is not the same as the volume of services available. However, where proportionate usage is very low the overall levels of service provision also tend to be relatively low, and in this respect seven of the above countries have both low coverage and low volume of formal services available (Bianchi, 1991; Hrynkiewicz *et al.*, 1991; Széman, 1992). In contrast, the other countries have usage of home-care services equal to or above the coverage of institutional care, and have a relatively high volume of services overall (Baro *et al.* 1991; Kraan *et al.*, 1991; Daatland, 1992).

Nevertheless, there does not appear to be a clear connection between levels of formal institutional care and home-care services. For example, Belgium, France and Finland each have approximately 5 per cent usage of institutional care by people aged over 65, but home-care usage of 5, 8 and 16 per cent respectively. However, what may be observed is that the lower the level of home-care the more likely it seems to be found alongside a lower level of institutional care. To understand the various approaches to the development of care services for older people, therefore, we must look separately to each type of provision. They also must be placed in context, within the shifting balance of what has come to be termed the 'welfare mix', in which the informal sector (usually family) as well as the formal state, market and voluntary (that is, non-profit-making) sectors each play a role (Huston, 1991; Evers and Svetlik, 1991). In particular, the debates about the forms of care provided have tended to concentrate on the opposition of institutional versus home-based care, and it is this divide which is shaping the form of service developments.

Institutional Life and Old Age

The rise of the institution

So, why are institutional forms of care under increasing criticism from many quarters? This can be explained partly by considering their history. In Europe, institutions derive, along with some other forms of welfare, from public responses to the relief of poverty. Variously described as 'almshouses', 'poor houses', 'workhouses' or 'houses of correction' depending on their formal purposes, the early institutions had in common that they represented a response by orderly society to destitution (de Beauvoir, 1977; Davis, 1981; Rusica *et al.*, 1991). They may be said to have reached their zenith in the nineteenth and twentieth centuries, reflecting wider forms of social structure. As factories came to constitute the pattern of industrial organisation, congregating workers in larger numbers under systematic control and segregating different types of work and stages in the process of production, so institutional forms of care became modelled on the lines of the factory. This can be seen in the growth and development of asylums and infirmaries, along with prisons and workhouses, and with the separation of 'deserving' from 'undeserving'; of 'mad' from 'bad' or 'sad'; and of these elements of life physically and socially from ordinary residence (Nirje, 1976; Foucault, 1977; Scull, 1979).

It is from this background that we can see the emergence of the institution in the care of older people (Clough, 1981; Giori, 1983; Guillemard, 1983; Means and Smith, 1985; Daatland, 1992). This heritage brings with it two underlying features which run through contemporary discussions. First, institutional care is provided for those who cannot make other arrangements. It is culturally and socially constructed as a 'last resort', of final choice or of no choice, at all. Second, institutions are focused on the common connection between the residents (their need for care) and not on degrees of individuality which may distinguish them. People are there because they are old (or have mental health problems, or learning disabilities and so on). The process of increased specialisation has tended to separate these service-user groups in recent times, but not everywhere, however – in Italy or Yugoslavia, for example, some areas may continue to provide for all groups of people in need in the same institution (Giori, 1983; Bianchi, 1991; Rusica *et al.*, 1991). The most general common factors shared by all these groups are that they have dependency needs of some kind and are likely to be poor.

These two features are both profoundly negative in their connotations for the social value that is placed on institutions. Under such circumstances it is hardly surprising that contemporary criticisms have been widespread and frequently vociferous, or that the social policies of many countries in recent decades have questioned institutional patterns of care. The negative standing of the institution affects the level and patterns of funding, and the education and training of the staff employed in them, as well as the status of the residents.

A fairly common criticism of some long-term residential provision for older people is that it is medically dominated, even when the need is for care rather than acute medical treatment (Kraan *et al.*, 1991). However, even when provision is defined as social rather than health, there may be some features which are the same, such as the ordering of daily routine or the use of space to suit the requirements of staff rather than the older people (Booth, 1985). Nor are all health facilities necessarily run in this way.

One solution to this aspect of the problem of 'institutionalisation' is in residential units which are defined as 'homes' rather than 'hospitals' or 'clinics'. These are to be found in some form in every European country (von Ballusek, 1983; Daatland, 1983 and 1992; Hunter, 1986; Lobo *et al.*,

1990; Carroll, 1991; Henrard, 1991). However, there are differences in the extent to which they are regarded as a health or a social service. The boundaries between nursing and social care (discussed briefly in the previous chapter) in practice will depend on national policies and the pattern of relationships between the various professions involved. Both types of care may be provided by the same type of home (as in France and Poland), or in very different types of home (as in Czechoslovakia, Denmark, Germany, Greece, The Netherlands, Norway, the UK and Yugoslavia). In some countries nursing care is provided solely within hospitals while residential homes as such only provide social care (as in Belgium, the Irish Republic, Finland, Hungary, Italy, Spain and Sweden).

From this it can be seen that there is no clear connection between the designation of types of care and the types of institutional arrangement that have been developed to provide them. State ownership or direct control of institutional services for older people has been prevalent in some parts of Europe, such as Scandinavia, the UK and Eastern Europe (although this is changing rapidly, for different reasons). In all European countries there is now a mix of state, voluntary (non-governmental, non-profit-making) and private-market agencies providing institutional care (Evers and Svetlik, 1991).

National variations

To explain these national differences in the use of, and developing social policies towards, institutional care for older people it is necessary to refer both to the history of welfare in each country as well as to the prevailing cultural expectations in the present. For the 'Mediterranean rim' countries of Greece, Italy (particularly the south), Portugal and Spain, and the Eastern European countries of Hungary, Poland and Yugoslavia, the late development of the welfare state and the rural/agricultural base of much economic and social life together appear to account for the relatively small scale of institutional care; it is also ascribed to the continuing power of family ideologies (Nazareth, 1976; Midre and Synak, 1987; Hrynkiewicz *et al.*, 1991; Jani-Le Bris, 1992; Stathopoulos and Amera, 1992).

At the other end of the spectrum, however, the larger-scale provision of residential care in the Irish Republic or The Netherlands are examples not of a lack of family care or – in the Irish Republic especially – of urban life. Rather strong social support for a welfare state in the late 1940s combined with the limited development of alternatives, derived from the dominance of specific professions within the formal service sectors, to concentrate care services in communal settings (Carroll, 1991; Nies *et al.*, 1991).

The common feature of these two extremes (which is also applicable to other countries) is that the extent of institutional care for older people appears to be related more to particular histories of welfare state development than to contemporary family structures or wider social ideologies.

Another possible factor underlying the numbers of older people using specific types of institutional care can be seen in the extent of state support for costs. In all countries, long-term residential care is means tested, with automatic state support for people with incomes assessed as being below the minimum (Evers and Svetlik, 1991; Kraan *et al.*, 1991). Only in Poland have residential homes for some time been formally free of charge (Hrynkiewicz *et al.*, 1991). However, the actual extent of support can directly affect the extent to which an individual can exercise choice. Again, Scandinavian countries are more comprehensive in their scale of support for the costs of institutional care, while this is more limited in countries such as Greece, Italy, Portugal or Spain (Bianchi, 1991; Stathopoulos and Amera, 1992).

In considering the proportions of older people receiving institutional care, it is necessary also to examine the age range of residents. A recent review of Scandinavian policy and practice draws attention to the bias towards its use by people over the age of 80 years (Daatland, 1992). These figures vary from 19 per cent in Denmark, through 22 per cent in Norway and Sweden to 28 per cent in Finland, in comparison to the over 65 figures noted on page 125 above, of 5 to 9 per cent (Daatland, 1992, p. 42). Similar data are evident for EC countries, and this phenomenon is related to the increased levels of disability in older old age which were noted in previous chapters (Jani-Le Bris, 1992). This suggests a close link with the possibility that other services might be able to provide appropriate levels of care more readily for younger old people, or that families might contribute a level of care comparable to formal, home-based services, but that neither can cope beyond a certain point of dependence – which is more likely to be reached in advanced old age. I will return to this question later in this chapter. First I want to consider why institutional care for older people has been so heavily criticised in recent years, especially as it occupies a major place in the range of social responses; and then to look at ways in which it is being reformed.

Challenges to institutions

The very term 'institutional' has ceased to be merely descriptive and has taken on a value-laden pejorative tone. My inclusion of residential homes within the concept of institutional care will therefore be heavily coded for

some readers, to say the least. 'Institutional' has become not only a cat-
egorical ascription but also (and sometimes at the same time) a critique.

The central theorist in this development has been Goffman (1968) who
proposed the concept of the 'total institution' to describe communal living
contexts in which certain features of social organisation could be identified.
These features include the separation of residents literally or symbolically
from the rest of society; limiting or denying their individuality; concentrat-
ing all aspects of life in one place; and staff control of the use of time and
space by residents (Goffman, 1968, p. 17). This led, in Goffman's terms, to
the 'mortification of the self'; that is, to the forcible erasure of the person-
hood of the resident by the pattern of life in the institution. This analysis
has evoked powerfully the comparison of institutional care with other
forms of communal life (particularly those in which choice of residence is
limited or non-existent), and the use of terms such as 'inmate' to describe
residents or 'internment' to describe the process of admission, reinforce the
sense that old people's homes and hospitals have more in common with
prisons or the poor-house than they do with an ordinary family home (see,
for example, de Beauvoir, 1977; Giori, 1983).

Evidence from a wide variety of research literature gives graphic
accounts of the types of practice which have fuelled criticisms. In the UK,
for example, these have included forcible bathing of new residents, regi-
mented mealtimes, a lack of personal clothing, a general lack of privacy
(such as the lack of locks on toilet doors, use of commodes in dormitories
and so on) and denigratory language used by staff towards residents
(Fennell *et al.*, 1988). In Hungary, residents have had to give up personal
possessions (Széman and Sik, 1991). In Italy, Bianchi (1991) observes, the
cleaning of rooms and cleaning of people have often been treated with the
same lack of finesse. It is clear from de Beauvoir (1977), de Campos
(1980), Giori (1983), Booth (1985), Dieck (1990) and Triantafillou and
Mestheneos (1990) that these criticisms are not confined to Hungary, Italy
or the UK, and that the practices to which they refer may have continued
for some time. It appears to be a shared experience that institutional care
has so often led older people into a state of 'acquired incompetence' (Evers
and Olk, 1991, p. 79).

Not only have there been critical research studies, but professionals and
policy makers have also addressed this issue. I noted above (see page 128)
the impact of Danish and Swedish psychologists through their development of the principle of 'normalisation' in services for people with learning difficulties, which proposes the use of culturally valued means to
provide care so that service users themselves are not devalued (Bank-
Mikkelson, 1976; Nirje, 1976). This has contributed to the more wide-

spread and growing preferences for non-instititutional care, because it identifies the way in which institutions themselves are bound up inexorably with the actions of staff as well as of residents.

These professional criticisms are having a marked impact on thinking about the care of older people (de Campos, 1980; von Ballusek, 1983; Giori, 1983; Booth, 1985; Fennell *et al.*, 1988). Consequently, it may be unjust to continue to refer to this research as if it necessarily describes all contemporary residential care. Changes in policy and practice have been engendered in part as a direct response to the exposure of the minutiae of institutional life and their effects to a wider public scrutiny. These changes can be divided broadly into those which propose a reform of institutional care in new models of communal life and those which dispense altogether with shared living as the basis of care. Let us look first of all at some of the ways in which the reform of communal care for older people has been developed in an attempt to overcome the implications of institutionalism.

Breaking down the walls?

One major objection to institutional living is that it produces impersonal care by restricting social contact between residents and people outside. Any attempts to reform communal care would have to address the issue of social relationships and links with ordinary life in the outside community. There are two ways in which this is being pursued.

The first of these is the development of greater flexibility of life in residential homes, enabling residents to have greater control over their lifestyle and to pursue relationships with people outside. In France and the UK this has been sought in some places through the development of links with community groups such as social clubs, churches and other organisations, or else through the encouragement of elderly residents to maintain friendships and family ties and for family members to participate in caring (Willcocks, 1982; Willcocks *et al.*, 1987; Pitaud and Vercauteren, 1991). In Germany, The Netherlands and Sweden the more radical step of restructuring long-term care as intensive congregate housing has encouraged older people and their younger relatives and friends to regard facilities as more like ordinary living (Fogarty, 1986; Kraan *et al.*, 1991).

The other way in which institutions can be opened up to the community is through the provision of services to people who are not actually resident (Davis, 1982; Willcocks, 1982). Examples may be seen in Greece, where residential homes may provide rehabilitation services for people living locally (Stathopoulos and Amera, 1992) and in The Netherlands where a wide range of services including meals, bathing and alarm systems are available from residential centres (Kraan *et al.*, 1991). Day-care in residential units exists in Germany, The Netherlands, the Scandinavian countries and the UK (Fogarty, 1986; Hunter, 1986). As yet, this flexibility is not evident in Eastern Europe, although the potential is recognised (Hartl, 1991; Széman and Sik, 1991).

However, this is a contentious use of such facilities because to the extent that day-care opens up the residential unit to the community, this may prove to be disruptive to the long-stay residents and operate counter to their rights to stability and privacy (Willcocks *et al.*, 1987). The recent review of residential care in the UK proposed that where day-care is provided in the same premises as residential care there should be a separation (for example, through a different entrance) and that long-stay residents who wish to make use of the separate service should be enabled to do so as a distinct activity (Wagner, 1990). This addresses Goffman's point about institutionalising use of space, as in this model the elderly resident 'goes out' and 'comes home again' in the same way as the person who lives in his or her own home, and s/he does not have someone else coming 'into his/her home' as a day centre. There seems to be very little evidence that this question has been given much consideration in any part of Europe, as for the most part concern is focused more on how to extend the range of services with static levels of resource.

Changes inside institutions

Concern with the social and psychological implications of size, the use of space and physical layout has also developed as a means of countering institutionalisation within residential care for older people .

The question of size is exemplified by movements in Scandinavia and the UK to establish 'small group living' arrangements, as subdivisions of larger units or by constructing smaller 'home-like' facilities (Willcocks, 1982; Willcocks *et al.*, 1987; Kraan *et al.*, 1991). The concept behind these facilities is to break up an institutional context into small groups of older people, usually numbering between six and ten. This size, it is argued, will enable patterns of relationship and action to develop which are more domestic in scale. The possibility of personal relationships developing is enhanced (Gupta, 1979; Peace, 1982). It is notable that such developments are located in the northern countries with the higher levels of institutional provision. This may be the result of greater experience, or else it may be a pragmatic compromise of deinstitutionalising services while maintaining the use of existing facilities.

However, in many countries the provision of single bedrooms and rooms for couples is the more urgent policy objective, and in many instances this remains a goal rather than an accomplishment (Fogarty, 1986; Evers and Svetlik, 1991). Changes in the types of building used for old people's homes, or adaptations of existing provision to create more private space and greater accessibility, may be said broadly to be a common European policy. However, the available resources and hence the underlying capacity to make this a reality are not spread evenly between countries; they are concentrated in the north and the west.

In the UK, Booth (1985) also questioned the impact of different care regimes of residential homes on the levels of dependency among older people. This research, which looked at 175 homes with total of 6954 residents over a three-year period (Booth, 1985, p. 31), concludes that 'the outcomes of care are not related to the way homes are run, or to current notions of good and bad practice' and raises the question again of whether institutional care should be provided at all (Booth, 1985, p. 219). Booth is writing here not only about measurable indices of dependence but also about those observable actions and arrangements which contribute to the meeting of 'codes of practice' concerning the rights of residents, including the question of who defines rights and who writes the codes.

That less institutionalised regimes do not produce diminished levels of dependence should not be surprising. The concept of institutional neurosis and other ideas about the negative effect of communal life on individuals are referring to behaviour and personality as opposed to 'measurable dependence'. In addition, it can be argued that it may be more acceptable for older people to live within non-institutional regimes simply on the grounds that they do have their rights respected (Foster, 1991). What may be of greater concern is the linked finding that many older people do not need the levels of care provided in a residential setting, but are there for lack of alternatives. This is apparent from research in the Irish Republic, France, The Netherlands and Sweden as well as the UK (Fogarty, 1986; Thorslund and Johansson, 1987; Carroll, 1991; Nies *et al.*, 1991). As Isaacs and Neville (1976) showed, in research undertaken in Scotland, care needs arising from disability or infirmity seldom if ever require the 24-hours-a-day response inherent in residential contexts, and these are the predominant dependency needs among older people. If the purpose of care is to meet these needs it should be structured in such a way as to do just that and no more, both on the grounds of cost and of minimising the intrusion of care into the lives of older people. The choice to live in a group context would then be based on different reasons, for example, as a means of ensuring companionship.

In those countries with a low base of institutional care, such as Greece, Hungary, Poland, Portugal and Spain, policy remains committed to the development of residential care for older people (Hrynkiewicz *et al.*, 1991; Széman and Sik, 1991; Anderson, 1992; Stathopoulos and Amera, 1992). It is argued that there are still many older people who are not able to live independently with dignity and for whom a degree of institutional care will be necessary. At present, therefore, these countries look set to increase the levels of formal residential care, even though available evidence shows the extent to which residential care in all countries is regarded by older people and their families as a last resort (Széman and Sik, 1991; Allen *et al.*, 1992).

It may be suggested that in Europe as a whole there is ambivalence about institutional contexts. That there seem to be limited possibilities of changing them while at the same time there is widespread questioning of the reasons for their perpetuation leads to the conclusion that institutional provision should be provided only to those for whom there is no other viable care. For all other older people care should be provided in ordinary domestic contexts. It should be 'at home' instead of 'in a home' to the greatest feasible extent, and this means community care.

In the Community

Where is the community?

'Community care' for older people in some guise is high on policy and professional agendas throughout Europe, as well as in Australia, Canada, the USA (Bulmer, 1987; Daatland, 1992). This may, as we have just seen, be in response to an historical critical focus on institutions, or it may, as in the 'Mediterranean rim' and Eastern Europe, be in recognition of family care as the historical norm and the very limited development of alternatives (Synak, 1987b; Dontas *et al.*, 1991). For some countries, therefore, community care policies may involve the transfer of resources into community-based contexts, while in others it may mean the development of these services as an addition to the development of institutions.

Bulmer, among others, has drawn attention to the multiplicity of definitions of 'the community' (Bulmer, 1987, pp. 26–35). It is now a common criticism within social science and elsewhere that the idea of community is strong on positive values but weak in relation to positive features by which it may be clearly identified. The community is an idea to which we can readily subscribe but in substance is difficult to find. This may be because in relation to the care of older people (or other groups of people with dependency needs) the reality of community may simply be a euphemism for 'not in an institution'.

A different but related point is made by French social gerontologists, who note that concern with 'community care' is an 'Anglo-Saxon' definition of terms (for example, Henrard, 1991). It is argued that the issue is one of whether care is provided at home. The question of who provides the care is separated and seen as a matter of the form taken by 'social solidarities' (Pitaud and Vercauteren, 1991). By this they mean that it is an issue of *how* families and the state work together to provide care and support, and not *whether* they do so. As Jamieson (1991a, 1991b) notes, this does not mean that the relationship between institutional and home-based care is made simpler in policy or practice, but rather that it becomes more clearly defined as one in which the *home* base is the second dimension, rather than relying on the more abstract nature of the concept of community. For this reason the French policy is referred to as *maintien-à-domicile*.

However, this may reflect a difference of emphasis. Home nursing may be categorised as home-based care because it takes place in the older person's own home, whereas a day-hospital is not home-based in the same sense. The point is that the older person does not have to change residence in order to make use of it (see the discussion in Chapter 5), and this is the nub of the French argument. Similarly, the extent to which either may be community-based also depends on emphasis.

The former ties several aspects of life to the one setting (the home), while the latter segregates people and puts them together in a batch (the day-hospital); both types of care apparently contain aspects of Goffman's concept of the 'total institution'. This suggests community by degrees, or else different communities according to circumstances. However, people who receive services at home are in the community in that they are in ordinary housing, with privacy, among family and friends and able to control their own use of time and space (within cultural norms); people who attend a day-hospital are also receiving help in a culturally normative manner, one which does not intrude into other aspects of their lives, and in that way are part of the wider community as compared to one defined by age or disability. Both may also be regarded as being part of a community of interest as older people who are using public services, in the sense that they thereby share some common elements of relationship to the wider society, the state and so on.

For most purposes, then, community care as it is reflected in contemporary European policies and practices means that which can be provided to older people who remain resident in their own homes as opposed to any more complex formulation which might consider the conceptual elements in the distinction between community and institution. Moreover, we might note also that the actual content of the care does not necessarily change between institution and community. Each type of service, whether it is meals-on-wheels, a social centre, home help, home nursing, day-care or day-hospital, provides something of the range of assistance provided by an institution. What is different is that it will be only that part which the older person requires or is judged by a third party (such as a professional) to need. In principle, this makes community care less costly as well as more flexible and more responsive to the older person.

The practice, however, may diverge from the principle quite markedly in some instances. The quality and quantity of services, especially as perceived by the individual service user, is not conveyed necessarily in a country by country review of what might be available (Jamieson, 1991b). There are regional disparities, demonstrated by national studies in Greece (Dontas, 1987; Amira, 1990); Italy (Giori, 1983; Bianchi, 1991); and the UK (Victor, 1987; Lawson *et al.*, 1991). Generally, there is a metropolitan concentration of resources for older people, which in some countries is less marked and takes the form more of an urban – rural divide (Henrard, 1991).

Moreover, not only is there a question concerning geographical equity in the distribution of community care services but also an issue around whether these are the correct services for the needs older people have, and who determines the basis of need, as well as doubts about the overall levels of service on a nation-by-nation basis (Kraan *et al.*, 1991). These are difficult questions to answer, not only because the definition of need is itself as much a social and political as a technical task (Bradshaw, 1972), but also because the large scale of family care disguises the extent to which public services might be required by older people themselves, or by their carers as an alternative or a supplement to informal caring (von Ballusek, 1983; Daatland, 1990; Siim, 1990). Jamieson (1991b) refers to a continuum of home-care policies, from those which are intended to substitute for informal care, through those which aim to complement and support informal carers, to those which provide a safety net for people without any potential informal care. The development of community care is therefore not only related to a criticism of and movement away from institutions but also concerns the role of the family and the role of older people themselves in providing care.

In, by or for the community?

If it can be said that there is not 'a community' of or for older people but rather several possible communities, to what extent do community-care policies address this diversity? Do such policies, for example, acknowledge the differences between the relationship patterns of specific families, do they recognise the implicit gender divisions of family life, and do they take into account the wider structural differences between families as these are affected by class or ethnic background?

In recent years there has been a growing body of critical appraisal of the reality of community care policies, especially in north and west Europe, which has both posed and provided answers to these questions. For the purposes of more detailed discussion, these critical approaches will be divided into two distinct groups, although there are in fact some overlaps between them.

The first of these addresses the implications of gender relations for the family care of older people. In what is now the classic formulation of the issue, Finch and Groves (1980) noted how policies and practices in the UK had gradually moved from care *in* the community to care *by* the community, and that this meant care by families. Moreover, the nature of the community was discovered not to be monolithic, but to be segregated on a number of dimensions, of which the most important in this regard is gender: in short, care by families actually means care by female relatives. So the subsequently published, quite explicit intention of the UK government to translate community care for older people into family care (DHSS, 1981) had already been shown to be inherently sexist.

This theme has also been addressed by critical studies in Germany and Scandinavia. The situation has been shown not only to relate to the extent of reliance on women to undertake caring tasks for elderly relatives but also in the extent to which women undertaking these tasks are likely to receive any type of public support. Wærness (1990) reviews research findings in Norway which point to the fourfold chance of a male carer (in the age group 64 to 75) receiving supportive services compared to a similar female carer. This situation also exists in Finland and Sweden, and Wærness suggests that, in common with Germany, the UK and North America, the patriarchy of the state shows through its responses to the family care of older people. In Denmark, Siim (1990) has argued that similar changes represent not so much an assertion of the patriarchal family values of the state as the re-emergence of such values after a period in which the state had tended to support women's interests. Denmark appears to be unique in this, and the Danish situation regarding the social expectation of women's roles within the family may explain partly the very full range of services available.

It is important to note that the gender inequalities of access to support services are seen among older carers because it is in the older, as opposed to the middle, age group that men are more likely to be carers, while the predominance of women as carers overall derives from the very large numbers of women in the 45 to 65 age range who are caring for elderly parents. Evidence from The Netherlands and the UK shows that elderly carers are most likely to be men caring for wives (Arber and Gilbert, 1989; Wenger, 1989; Parker, 1990; Pijl, 1991). However, a different picture emerges in Denmark, France, Germany, Greece, Italy and Sweden (Sundstrøm, 1986; Amira, 1990; Bianchi, 1991; Jani-Le Bris, 1992). In each of these countries studies suggest that women of all ages are more likely to be carers. Some national differences can be observed also in the use of formal support services. The conclusion reached by Arber and Gilbert (1989) in the UK was that there were no gender differences in support given to older carers, while Sundstrøm (1986) in Sweden and Wærness (1990) in Norway recorded gender biases (that is, men caring, or living alone, are more likely than women in similar circumstances to have available formal support services). However, the UK data included all older people, whereas the Scandinavian figures refer only to the younger group of older people (aged 64 to 75), so relative age may also be a factor.

The reality of gender divisions in community care, especially affecting younger carers, has led to calls for a change of both emphasis and direction in old-age welfare policies and practices. In Scandinavia, several analyses have suggested that it would be an advance for policy-makers to recognise the large extent to which family care is provided, to acknowledge the strengths of this and to offer appropriate support (Sundstrøm, 1986; Wærness, 1990; Johansson, 1991). At the same time the system would be improved by making family care a real choice, which could only be achieved through reconstructing residential care as a viable alternative (by overcoming problems of institutionalisation, which I discussed on page 132). This latter point has been made in more detail in the UK, where Finch (1984), Dalley (1988) and Foster (1991) have variously proposed residential care as the basis for overcoming sexism in this arena, given that they are pessimistic about the possibility of reform in the sexism of wider social structures. I will return to the implications of Scandinavian experience in the final chapter, as the emphasis there on the expansion of home-based care has clear gender implications.

The second area of discrimination in community care for older people is that of race and ethnic background. Several studies in the UK have demonstrated that despite some attempts to create relevant and acceptable services there remains a substantial degree of racism, whether overt or unintended (Torkington, 1983; Norman, 1985; Rooney, 1987). Not only do ethnic-minority service users face hostility or inappropriate responses on an individual level (such as questioning a person's entitlement to services, making false assumptions about levels of family support and so on), but there are problems of language, of culture and of general image. Community care services have not been widely promoted among ethnic minority communities, partly because of language barriers, but also because they have they have not always been, or been perceived as being, appropriate (Bhalla and Blakemore, 1981; Norman, 1985; Williams, 1990). Some other older, non-English-speaking white people have also suffered a lack of supportive services for the same reasons, including migrants from other European countries (Norman, 1985). Even attempts to provide appropriate services have not always been successful, as illustrated by problems with meals-on-wheels services which have failed to recognise the ethnic diversity between different groups (Rooney, 1987).

As discussed earlier, countries such as France, Germany and The Netherlands, like the UK, have a history of immigration from former colonies, and all European countries have some immigrants from non-European nations (de Jouvenal, 1988; Evers and Olk, 1991; Pijl, 1991). In this context, the integration of the former GDR (German Democratic Republic) with the FDR (Federal Republic of Germany) has implications of an internal 'colonisation', as the cultural differences in approaches to old age and care for older people were quite marked between the two halves of the now united country, even though there is a high degree of common ethnicity (Evers and Olk, 1991; Fischer, 1993).

It appears that all European countries will have some older members of ethnic minorities for whom care services will be required, yet this is an issue which is only just beginning to be addressed. The relatively small proportion of older people within ethnic minority communities makes them even less visible to white European policy-makers and professionals, so that they are further marginalised: a minority within minorities.

As with feminist criticism, anti-racist writers have argued for a shift in policy and practice. It is here that black control has been advocated as a desirable alternative in the UK, with the planning and implementation of home help, meals-on-wheels and other comparable services to be undertaken by black organisations for black service users on behalf of the state (Phillips, 1982; Norman, 1985; Rooney, 1987; Williams, 1990). Such groups, it is suggested, are able to recognise and respond appropriately to cultural requirements and to cope with diversity in a way that white dominated services are not.

The third area of discrimination relates to class. This is a question which is more widely acknowledged in European studies of community care for older people. Examples include evidence that older people who are more affluent make greater use of the open-care centres in Greece; that the direct costs of care have been shifted towards older people themselves or their families in Germany; and that in the UK it is the middle classes who have greatest access to the National Health Services (of which older people are the main users), or to private care services where there are fewer restrictions on access (Townsend and Davidson, 1982; von Ballusek, 1983; Victor, 1987; Dieck, 1990; Teperoglou *et al.*, 1990). The studies by Tentori (1976) and Bonanus and Calasanti (1986) in rural southern Italy show more generally how class has remained a key factor in the life of older people, not only affecting income and other material resources for coping in later life but also being related to family relationships and to the cultural means for adapting to old age. Social class is a major division between older people living in the same geographical community, which is related to differences in standard of life, the type and extent of care available and so on. Bianchi (1991) points to ways in which class plays a more subtle part in northern Italy, through means tests for public services and the existence of expensive private alternatives. Similar, quasi-class-related effects of inequalities in wealth are evident also in the Eastern European countries in the variations of access by older people to home-based as well as residential care services (Hartl, 1991; Széman, 1992).

So although the formal ideology behind the formation of state welfare services has often been to provide assistance for the poorer groups in society (Siim, 1990, p. 85), this does not appear to have changed the social advantages of the middle and upper classes. This is because the advantages which are exercised on a class basis are not only related to levels of income but also to the knowledge and patterns of action which are necessary to make the most effective use of community care services and primary health care. Critics have suggested that it is not only a matter of extending the quantity of services available (although that is part of the problem) but also of making the services more accessible (Elder, 1977; Bornat *et al.*, 1985). Means tests and other devices to ration services according to income may be stigmatising, and as those who are wealthy can purchase alternatives, often serve to deny community care to those older people who have relatively modest means but who are not classified as poor (Walker, 1986b and 1990). As Walker (1990) shows in relation to Germany, Norway and the UK, poverty is also likely to increase with advancing age and that this is related to types of previous employment and levels of pension income. In the Scandinavian countries generally there is a lower level of poverty in old age because the pension system has been based on transfer income, while in Germany the social insurance system 'can lead to an insufficient level of financial security' for elderly people (Evers and Olk, 1991, p. 63). As the former allows for the risk of care needs increasing while the latter does not,

German older people who need care are often likely to make a claim on the social assistance scheme.

The income dimension to social class divisions has been stressed because it is the major factor in the variation of access to community care and primary health services among older people. It is this factor also from which the interconnections between different forms of discrimination can be identified. That is, although any one of the dimensions which have been discussed – gender, race, ethnicity or class – affects the availability and the quality of community care, these are likely to occur in some combination rather than on their own. In the UK study by Bhalla and Blakemore (1981), social class combined with race in affecting the differential levels of community care provided to white European, Afro-Caribbean and Asian older people. Similarly Bryan *et al.* (1985) have argued that being a woman compounds the discrimination faced by being black in the availability of appropriate services. Greater poverty among women, whether as elderly people or as carers, has been shown to affect older women of all ethnic backgrounds (Walker, 1987; Evers and Olk, 1991; Pijl, 1991). Although each form of discrimination has a distinct impact, they come together in various ways to create situations of multiple discrimination (Norman, 1985). Moreover, all these discriminations are compounded in some sense by that of ageism, which is faced inescapably by all older people and their carers.

So there are different communities to which older people and their carers belong each, of which face similar and related but distinct sets of issues in constructing and responding to the demands of community care. The common themes are to be found in the difficulties encountered in levels of and access to appropriate services. This could be taken to suggest that families only provide care for elderly members because there is no alternative, but the discussion in Chapter 3 showed that across Europe as a whole there is still a strong ideology of family care. What is at issue for most critics of community care is the extent to which such services support families and provide open, flexible ranges of care from which older people can choose. The one possible exception to this is the feminist argument that under present circumstances it is not possible for community care to avoid sexism and that the development of high-quality residential or other communal alternatives should therefore become a priority. What would be the implications of this and other developments in the care of older people? Furthermore, to what extent are these issues of concern only in those parts of Europe in which institutional services have existed on a relatively large scale in the past? It is these questions I will address in the rest of this chapter.

Institutionalising the Community?

Dismantling, dispersing or transforming institutions?

It is possible to equate the enthusiasm in policy and practice for home-based or community care for older people with the theoretical criticisms of institutional life. However, it is necessary to consider the impact of such critiques alongside other factors in policy and practice developments. It has been noted above that there is a division in Europe between those countries in which home-based or community care is now advocated as an *alternative* to institutional provision, while in others it is seen as an *addition* to the development of residential care. This division roughly follows a north-west/south-east boundary separating countries with relatively high and low proportions of institutional care provision. However, the stress now placed on developing community care services for older people as a policy priority are as great in countries that already have very high levels of such provision (for example, Denmark, Finland, Norway and Sweden) as in those countries which are in the middle range (such as Belgium, France, Luxembourg, The Netherlands and the UK) (see Table 6.1 on page 125) (Kraan *et al.*, 1991). It is the countries with the lowest levels of home-care services that are also most likely to have policies which include the expansion of institutional care alongside community care (such as Greece, Hungary, Italy, Poland, Portugal and Spain) (Anderson, 1992). Only the Irish Republic and Germany have relatively low levels of home-care services, laying stress on community provision rather than institutional developments.

This suggests that the pressure for growth in home-based or community-care services does not spring solely from a rejection of residential provision. Jamieson (1991c) points to the differences between the Danish experience and that of The Netherlands or the UK in the extent to which a lack of home-care will result in greater demand for residential care rather than to more caring provided by family or other informal carers. In other words, in countries with already very high levels of community care (for example, Scandinavia) the pressure for even more comes from an established expectation that such care substitutes for both residential and informal care. In the countries with middle levels of community care (such as France, The Netherlands and the UK), developments are intended to expand the support available to informal carers and so limit the possible rise in demand for institutional provision. This would apply also to the Irish Republic and Germany. In all these countries the common threads are the projected rises in the numbers of older elderly people (those people most likely to need care support) and the greater costs to the state of formal versus informal care. In other words, this cannot be separated from the political economy of old age and social welfare (Svetlik, 1991; Daatland, 1992). The critique of institutions is harnessed to the political objective of reducing state involvement in direct welfare provision. So in those countries in the south and east with low levels of residential care we may expect to see a more rapid expansion of community care than is currently envisaged, as the fiscal crises of state welfare are experienced (Bianchi, 1991; Hartl, 1991; Stathopoulos and Amera, 1992). These are also the countries in which the ideology of direct family care remains strongest, and so policies to support rather than substitute for informal care, except at the residual level, might be expected.

The timing of a move away from institutional care is not only based on late-twentieth-century political economy: it is also possible in practice because alternative 'technologies' are now available (Foucault, 1977; Scull, 1984). Technologies in this sense not only mean the physical equipment which can now be utilised to support older people in non-institutional surroundings (such as alarm systems, intercoms, radio-pagers and so on) but also the organisational systems through which home-based and community-care services are provided. These include devolved management, the transfer of state funds to independent service providers and new professional practices (Jamieson, 1991c; Kraan *et al.*, 1991).

This is not to argue that the reality of life for older people using community care services has not changed. The presence of an alarm system through which assistance can be summoned may enable relatives, friends and professionals to feel more comfortable about a frail older person remaining in his or her own home and so reduce the pressure which they might feel to intervene or to seek residential care as a form of security. The effect of blurring institution and community arising from the increased surveillance inherent in electronic monitoring may be a price worth paying for the choice to remain at home – for the whole of society as well as for the individual. However, it must be recognised that there is a social as well as an economic cost, in that technology may make it easier for older people to become subject to inappropriate surveillance or monitoring in the name of appropriate concern. The dilemma is in maintaining the right of older people to make informed judgements about the risks they face (Norman, 1980).

Transformations of institutional care may also be achieved in the same way. The 'group living' concept in residential homes discussed earlier represents just such a movement, as does the creation of small residential units, in which issues of scale and segregation are challenged through an explicit engineering of the living environment. Here, again, physical and social technologies play a part in enabling social controls over dependence to be maintained while promoting greater individual dignity and privacy among older people themselves.

To what extent should we follow the argument that the move from residential to community care, to whatever degree, does not dismantle the institution but transforms it in ways which potentially enhance the power of the state and professionals over older people? This can be seen as a process of 'institutionalising the community'. The weakness of this critical argument can be seen in its focus on mental health and criminal justice as the central models of social control. The care of older people, it could be suggested, is not comparable to these issues. This is true to the extent that 'dependence' is not the same as 'deviance' (and that mental ill-health has so often been regarded as the latter rather than the former). However, historically, institutions have not always distinguished between the two. Typically they were managed in such a way as to stress a concern with control as much as with care. In so far as institutionalisation has affected care for older people, the social processes of deinstitutionalisation may also be seen as relevant. Indeed, it is the same physical and social technologies that enable it to occur, and in a country such as Italy, where deinstitutionalisation is high on the political and professional agenda, common cause is made between older people and people with mental health problems or learning difficulties (Giori, 1983; Bianchi, 1991).

Reformation of residential care as a feminist project has a different origin, namely the critique of community care in Scandinavia and northern Europe (Finch, 1984; Sundstrøm, 1986; Siim, 1990; Wærness, 1990; Foster, 1991). It sets out the agenda not so much in terms of asking in what ways might institutions be transformed, but rather by stating that a way must be found to transform residential care as the best non-sexist option. Inasmuch as 'the family' equates with women relatives, then the social cost of community care for older people is discriminatory.

The critique of institutional care and the critique of community care for older people would seem, therefore, to be in a contradictory relationship. Both are pertinent analyses of the contemporary situation, but they come to exactly opposite conclusions.

A resolution of this contradiction may lie in the possibility for the exercise of choice by older people themselves, at the same time as informal carers are also enabled to exercise choice: in other words, to create situations in which the older person can choose whether or not to enter a residential home without the opportunity to stay at home being reliant on the caring work of a daughter, daughter-in-law or other relative. Research evidence suggests that high proportions of older people in residential care were satisfied with this assistance, and that relief of loneliness was a major factor. Figures include 73 per cent in the UK and 66 per cent in Hungary (Széman and Sik, 1991; Allen *et al.*, 1992), and loneliness appears to have been the major factor in admissions. However, such research also reveals widespread comments which suggest a reluctance to complain, because there was nowhere else suitable to live, or because of the perceived burden on relatives. The preferences shown in many countries for different forms of supported accommodation do suggest also that the 'last resort' view of residential care, even if it is found to be acceptable, is widely shared across Europe (Fogarty, 1986; Daatland, 1990).

Constructing the community

Patterns of community care which are intended to promote the degree of choice which can be exercised by older people through improved co-ordination of services at the individual or the operational level have been developed in The Netherlands and in the UK, and the lack of such co-ordination in other countries is regarded as being a key issue for the future (Hunter, 1986; Kraan *et al.*, 1991; Nies *et al.*, 1991). In both these countries the new patterns of co-ordination were until very recently to be found only in experimental projects, and were implemented as formal policies in the UK as recently as 1993. They are still in the process of being implemented in The Netherlands.

The Dutch approach has been to create projects managed by specialist social workers which bring together a range of community-based support services. In contrast the UK projects are based around the co-ordination of disparate services to individuals, also by specialist social workers acting as 'case managers' (Challis and Davies, 1986; Challis *et al.*, 1988). Three factors are central to the UK experiment with case management:

1. The projects were targeted at older people who were likely to enter residential care;
2. The case managers had direct control over specified budgets for some services and a responsibility to initiate integration with others; and
3. The case managers were responsible for the recruitment and management of non-professional carers.

The research findings are that these projects achieved the aim of helping older people to remain in their own homes where they wanted this, and also providing relief and support to family carers (Challis *et al.*, 1988; Davies and Missiakoulis, 1988).

These projects have been influential in that an adapted model of case management has been incorporated recently into UK legislation concerning community care, although some problems have been perceived in implementing the concept outside the bounds of experimental projects (DoH, 1990; Kubisa, 1990; Allen *et al.*, 1992). In particular, limitations on resources in some areas have been identified, as well as a lack of clarity in professional roles, plus difficulties in establishing co-operative links between social and health services (Challis, 1990; Allen *et al.*, 1992). Moreover, these schemes have been criticised because, by using non-professional carers outside normal employment procedures, it can be argued that the flexibility of the experimental projects was gained at the expense of women workers, who were paid at very low rates and had no employment security (Finch, 1984; Ungerson, 1990). It is argued that to be non-exploitative such work should be within normal employment patterns. Ungerson (1990) notes that this should not be expected to produce inappropriate relationships between carers and older people, and that interpersonal warmth (caring *about*) can be seen also in formal care contexts.

Such a view is supported by evidence from the policy development in Sweden of payment to informal carers at a 'full' wage-rate (Johansson, 1991). Family members can be 'employed' as home carers, to work solely with their elderly relative and have benefits such as paid holiday and support from other home-care services. This policy is aimed at increasing both the proportion and the total volume of informal care for older people as the numbers of older people grow. However, the Swedish evidence also shows that paid informal carers gave more time than the hours for which they were employed. Wider support for informal caring remains patchy, and its importance has not been widely grasped (Hokenstad and Johansson, 1990). Because of this, older people themselves and their families are being expected to meet the cost directly, rather than it being seen as a shared social obligation (Daatland, 1992).

Placing the responsibility for the direct cost of support and assistance on to individual older people occurs in the many forms of private sheltered-housing schemes which have proliferated in recent decades, especially in Northern Europe. Although some of these are provided through agencies which are non-fee-charging at the point of use, many more are privately owned on a condominium basis and there have even been a small number of successful 'retirement villages' established, although the majority of older people appear not to favour this type of segregation either (Fogarty, 1986). Such an approach is based on the assumption that most older people have accumulated resources during their lives, either in property (such as a house in countries where house-owning is normal) or in pensions. The provision of private domiciliary and community-care services are attached, sometimes at an additional cost. The principle behind such developments is that of consumerism: social control exercised through the power of the purchaser which enables the individual to make choices, which is appearing in a range of welfare contexts (Garland, 1990; Hugman, 1994). The flexibility and personal control afforded by the direct purchase of community care, either individually or through a housing scheme, does enhance the positive social value which can be placed on the use of services, and potentially minimises the stigma of dependence. The very concept of control over a situation is incompatible with the idea of being dependent. It means also that older people do not have to rely on their families for care support, either financially or practically.

There are two weaknesses to this consumerist model of community care. First, it assumes that the older person has access to the necessary resources to meet the costs. In other words, it carries with it implications about social class (which were discussed earlier), because class creates the material circumstances in which the private accumulation of the means (whether material, personal health or social resources) which shape the basis for the experience of old age can take place. Such resources are not available across the whole of European society but only to quite specific communities, defined on a social-class basis. Research comparing ten EC countries identified the reality of life for many older people as one of poor housing which does not provide the basis for a consumer revolution in care (Fogarty, 1986). For example, as many as 72 per cent of older people in one Italian city were living in housing conditions with poor facilities, and the figure of 77 per cent owner-occupiers in the Irish Republic 'should not be taken to indicate gracious living' (Fogarty, 1986, pp. 31–2). The costs of moving and the relatively high prices of private supported accommodation, as well as cultural attitudes towards housing change in old age, all act to set limits on this possibility.

Second, the consumerist concept assumes that older people are both well-informed and have the social power to act on information. Such an assumption ignores the extent to which people who are dependent on others may have a conflict of interest, or that their knowledge and preferences can be manipulated by those on whom they are dependent (Hugman, 1991). Professionals may not recognise that they possess information which older people need, older people may be placed or moved to suit the organisational interests of paid carers (even where the older person is directly fee-paying), or pressure from family members may influence older people in making decisions without fully considering all the implications (Tester and Meredith, 1987; Dieck, 1990; Hokenstad and Johansson, 1990; Lobo *et al.*, 1990).

Case management, the payment of family carers and retirement housing represent different approaches to thinking about claims on 'the community' as a basis for providing more flexible care for older people. Each takes aspects of community, seen in terms of the connections between residence and social relationships, and seeks to integrate flexible levels and types of care while responding to individuality and capacity for choice. All three can be said to have had at least limited success on these grounds. At the same time, case management and the payment of family carers can be said to share some of the problems which were previously identified, in so far as neither addresses the structural social divisions of gender (in the family or the community). The latter incorporates social class divisions in that it is dependent on access to sufficient income, and these carry with them implications of other inequalities, such as gender, race, ethnicity and disability. Age structures may also be a factor, in that people just into retirement years (late sixties and early seventies) form a sizeable body of voluntary assistance, so that localities with large proportions of 'younger' older people may be able to offer a wider range of supportive services to the smaller group of older people with dependency needs (Fogarty, 1986). Private sheltered housing schemes may therefore be inclined to recruit on age-related grounds and exclude older elderly people.

Regional variation and common concerns

The exact route taken by each country, or regions within countries, in balancing institutional and community-based care for older people varies according to historical, political, economic and cultural factors as each of these finds expression in social policy. Detailed policies of the combination of health and social provision, of formal and informal care, of the state and independent providers, reflect local conditions. It is not possible, ultimately, to produce a typology which takes all factors into account at the level of fine detail.

There is one common feature shared by all these countries, however. There is a connection between the growth in the number of older people, especially in the age range over 75 years (on whom welfare spending is highest in all European Community and Scandinavian states, for example) and ideological shifts in public policy towards individualisation and privatisation, which are driven by economic considerations (de Jouvenal, 1988; Svetlik, 1991). There has been a breakdown in consensus about the way in which care and assistance should be provided for those older people who need it, and how this should be financed. So all countries are seeking to expand community-based care, especially informal (family) care, irrespective of whether this is accompanied by a growth in or a reduction of institutional provision.

To that extent, the question of whether the issue of deinstitutionalisation is more or less relevant in any one part of Europe is perhaps less important than asking if ways can be found to develop the necessary community-based alternatives in which social as well as economic costs are taken fully into account. This distinction is crucial because, as debates within the feminist critique of community care have shown, the inter-generational aspect of pressures on families arising from community care can create hierarchies of discrimination (Finch and Groves, 1982; Morris, 1992). In defending the rights of women to chose whether or not to be carers, for example, there is a risk that elderly people are reconstructed as a 'burden', so playing into the new ageism – a key feature of the so-called 'age war' that is developing in North America as well as in Europe (Gruman, 1978; Estes, 1986; de Jouvenal, 1988; Johnson and Falkingham, 1992).

For these reasons it is possible to see common concerns in otherwise varied European countries, in responses to those older people who have care needs. However, in his summary of evidence from case studies of open (that is, community) care systems, Amann (1980b) concluded that social and political diversity should always be regarded as indicating differences between countries in the appropriateness of specific welfare programmes. He refers to the 'stages of development continuum' developed by Little (1979), which I examined in Chapter 5, as an explanatory concept (Amann, 1980b, p. 182). As was noted previously, this continuum was not intended by Little to be an evolutionary theory suggesting that countries would necessarily follow a particular pattern, but rather one to enable a multidimensional cross-national analysis of care for older people. This is emphasised by Amann's later critical comments concerning the inconsistencies of social security and social welfare systems in Western Europe and Scandinavia, and levels of institutionalisation in The Netherlands, although he subsequently eulogises Sweden as a model for community care (Amann, 1980b pp. 183, 193). More recent comparative data have showed the difficulties emerging from the rapid pace of political, economic and social change, and revealed a number of problems in taking any one country as a model for others as if, despite the caveats, there is a specific evolutionary trend which might produce the most desirable outcome (Jones, 1985; Evers and Svetlik, 1991). Indeed, Amann is aware of this and points to problems of comparison over time, including the future possibility that services such as home helps will be looked at askance in relation to the conditions which will then prevail. Moreover, care must be taken not to consider the transfer of experience only in one direction, towards those parts of Europe which have more lately moved towards welfare-state provision, rather than an approach based on a more mutual exchange of ideas.

From this cautionary standpoint it appears possible, nevertheless, to begin to consider how the development of welfare programmes might be informed by the experiences in other countries, and what degree of transferability is feasible within Europe as whole. Attempts to construct community care in parallel with institutional care development may have much to show those areas where the focus is on deinstitutionalising services. In the final chapter I want to turn to a discussion of specific case examples of changes taking place and recent programmes in the care of older people, as well as look at some problems which are to be faced in the future in Europe.

7
Europe: An Ageing Society

Old Age in the New Europe

The ageing enterprise

Welfare responses are expressions of the social values attaching to old age as much as of the material infrastructure within which old age is experienced. Any structured social response to ageing necessarily combines images of older people with ideas about the rights, needs and contributions of older members of society. Guillemard (1983, p. 93) has called this the 'cultural model of old age', which brings together social structures and relationships within an ethical framework. That is to say, welfare responses act as a vehicle for value systems and at the same time serve to provide an arena in which those values are shaped, remodelled and possibly even challenged. The example which Guillemard gives of this from the French context is of the increasing proportions of older middle-class people for whom the charitable image of need in old age was increasingly inappropriate, (this was discussed in Chapter 1), leading to an 'identity crisis' in the prevailing cultural model of ageing (Guillemard 1983, p. 95; also see Pitaud and Vercauteren, 1991, p. 35).

For this reason, the demographic changes taking place across Europe have to be understood in relation not only to the possible implications for the levels of services provided to those older people with dependency needs (quantity) but also the types of service (quality), especially in so far as they create and sustain images of old age. Not only, as we have seen, does this mean that previous institutional forms of care (in the critical analytic sense discussed in Chapter 6), with their deep connotations of poverty and charity, are increasingly unacceptable, but also that images of ordinariness and normality gain in power as the ideological force behind reform. Although the purchasing power of older people – old age as a consumer identity – plays a part, there is the complementary question of how this affects concepts of fairness and equity, both between generations and between distinct groups of older people (Dieck, 1990; Pitaud and Vercauteren, 1991).

It is patently inequitable for divisions of gender, race, ethnicity or class to determine the basis on which old age is defined. So we are left with the question, for example, that if a residual institutional state service is not appropriate for one group of older people should it be acceptable for another, and if not, how is equity to be maintained? It is in this way that the debates about community care in old age are tied to the relationship of social structure, demography, social value and patterns of welfare. As staying in one's own home as one gets older is the preference of most older people in all European countries, for a variety of reasons, it is vital that developing policies and practices should enable this to happen. This will not be achieved if the degree of choice it is possible to exercise (for example, between home-based care and residential care) is based on whether the older person is a woman or a man, on level of income, or on ethnic identity.

Within the European Community as it exists during the 1990s there is, as yet, only the start of a co-ordinated development of policies and practices to address these questions (Council of Europe, 1991b). To some extent this slow pace is not only inevitable but also desirable. As we have seen in previous chapters, there is a social and cultural diversity to old age in Europe which would make too narrow or too rapid a definition of policies and practices both unworkable and unwelcome. Nevertheless, the extent to which there are common issues of demography, economy and changing social relationships between European countries (many of which are already being addressed at a formal level) underlines the conclusion that at a European level the phenomenon of ageing and the care which is provided to older people has not only become essential but will increasingly be unavoidable.

The constitution of Europe is also changing through the emergence of a 'new Europe' following the collapse of the 'state socialist' regimes in Eastern European countries (Deacon, 1992a and 1992b). There are some very real problems to be encountered by older people, as pensions are being tied to the real level of wages (and so *falling*) for example, although in some countries, such as Czechoslovakia and Hungary, the impact is being offset by the retention of protected rents or housing subsidies for pensioners (Deacon, 1992b, pp. 100–1). At the same time, the trend to protect the corporatist health services appears to be being maintained in all the Eastern countries, even where either voluntary (usually the church) or private (profit making) sectors are being encouraged to develop.

At this early stage it is not possible to know which specific aspects of particular welfare services will follow the Western capitalist pathways, or indeed which variant of Western models (Pflanczer and Bognár, 1989; Deacon, 1992a). Even in the more 'Westernised' countries such as Czechoslovakia and Hungary the levels of provision may still be very low compared to assessed need (Pflanczer and Bognár, 1989; Hartl, 1991).

Possibilities for the future could include not only a progression towards the market mechanism models which are currently dominating Western Europe, even in countries with national health and social services systems, but also the potential for a move in the direction of the Scandinavian type of corporate public welfare. To a large extent the immediate possibilities were established by the way in which the previous systems actually operated, as opposed to their formal policies. The example of Hungary suggests that where the formal health and pension system failed to provide the level of support intended, and there is no residual private or charitable sector, then market forces may be seen as the most viable model to follow (Pflanczer and Bognár, 1989; Széman and Sik, 1991; Széman and Gáthy, 1993). The limitations of the more corporatist model in Scandinavia lie in the extent to which it can be sustained, a point to which I will return later in this chapter.

Concern to promote a European-wide policy on old age necessarily focuses on those issues on which a comparative position can be reached (Council of Europe, 1991b). It is feasible that in order to achieve any semblance of equality within an expanded European Community, the 'levelling of the playing field' will aim at a reasonably low common denominator (Deacon, 1992b, p. 105). Under these circumstances the interplay of social values with material relationships will be crucial, as the spread of systems of welfare in the EC already encompasses those that are very residualised (Germany) as well as those that are highly institutionalised within the state (Denmark) and many points in between (Pflanczer and Bognár, 1989). Will the common denominator be residual, or will it be more complex?

The idea of the 'welfare mix'

One way in which it has been suggested that the complexity of European policies and practices for older people can be grasped has been through the emergence of the idea of a 'welfare mix' (Rose and Shiratori, 1986; Evers and Wintersberger, 1988; Huston, 1991). Although this concept is primarily analytic, in that it does not describe a discrete approach, it does provide the basis for understanding that in all developed countries there are a number of 'social actors' involved in responding to the situation and needs of older people (Huston, 1991, p. 8). These actors are: the state; the market; private households (including families and older people themselves); and other independent groups (non-profit-making, non-government organisations). What the idea of the welfare mix brings to the understanding of social responses to older people is that it challenges the more rigid distinctions of the conservative/liberal/social democratic typology (Esping-Andersen, 1990).

Evers and Olk (1991) argue that the important questions in the analysis of welfare systems are those which concern the balances between different 'actors'. So the concentration in Germany of the role of the state in ensuring that welfare for older people is controlled and financed produces a particular mix, one which is grounded in 'liberal state traditions and Catholic social ethics' (Evers and Olk, 1991, p. 68). The German welfare state is therefore one which enables but does not directly provide care services. This is to be seen as a different mix from Denmark, The Netherlands, or the UK, in which the balance and roles of the different actors vary, and in which the greater role of the state as a provider is congruent with other political and cultural (including religious) traditions. This should then enable specific policies or practices to have an impact on a particular mix, rather than raising questions about whether it is or is not congruent with a welfare state type.

At the analytic level, therefore, the welfare mix concept is very useful. However, as we have seen in previous chapters, there may be concerns about its use to advocate shifts away from specific welfare state forms. In particular, the stronger traditions of direct state involvement in the provision of welfare for older people in northern Europe (Denmark, Finland, The Netherlands, Norway, Sweden and the UK) may be based in social democratic or socialist (and Protestant) histories. It is in these countries that attempts to move away from direct public welfare have generated the recognition of the likely impact on informal carers, especially women (Finch and Groves, 1980 and 1983; Green, 1988; Siim, 1990; Wærness, 1990; Phillipson, 1992). This concern has subsequently begun to be echoed in other parts of Europe which do not share the same political and cultural traditions (Dieck and Naegele, 1989; Jani-Le Bris, 1992; Stathopoulos and Amera, 1992). Where the concept of welfare mix might be used is to point to the already massive involvement of families as actors in care provision so that shifts in other areas can be understood as having a system impact. It would not be helpful to informal carers if the concept was used simply to justify efforts to reduce direct state provision. This would be more likely to reinforce, or even create, perceptions of older people as a 'burden'. Where families are faced with other pressures, such as changes in economic patterns with greater employment of women, there is evidence that this is happening, for example in the abandoning of elderly people at hospitals. This is beginning to occur in countries with strong traditions of family responsibility and honour as well as in those countries with long histories of state provision (Triantafillou and Mestheneos, 1990).

The ageing conflict

As I have discussed at several points in the preceding chapters, demographic trends have created a powerful upsurge of opinion which gives a novel twist to the crisis of cultural identity as it is defined by Guillemard (1983). Rather than wishing to promote old age as a stage of the life-cycle in which equality of opportunity and social access are a right of citizenship, as opposed to a period of dependence and withdrawal, old age is characterised as a form of consumption which is increasingly beyond our means (Callahan, 1986). The conclusion of this logic is that old people should not be 'favoured', as attempts to create greater equity are seen from this perspective, and that those who have not made private personal provision earlier in their lives should accept a right only to residual support (Dieck, 1990; Pitaud and Vercauteren, 1991). This type of argument has been widely criticised as a form of ageism (Giori, 1983; Estes, 1986; de Jouvenal, 1988; Wisensale, 1988; Dieck, 1990). A recognition of the potential social disruption arising from this perspective was part of the rationale in the designation of 1993 as 'European Year of Older People *and Solidarity Between the Generations*' (my emphasis) (Eurolink Age, 1992).

Johnson and Falkingham (1992, pp. 184–8) propose an alternative model of public welfare support for older people, recognising the underlying demands that may be placed on society in coming decades, but which avoids the trap of blaming or stigmatising particular social groups. This approach involves fixing income parity between wages and pensions, so establishing an equitable basis on which older people who are financially dependent are seen to do no better than other sections of society. There are two forms to this model. The first form is to relate the ratio of retirement pensions directly to earned income, a policy which has been pursued in parts of Scandinavia (Abrahamson, 1991), although Johnson and Falkingham suggest that this is less far-reaching because it remains ageist in its assumption of age-related eligibility. The other form is to create a single system of financial support for all non-wage-earners in a basic income scheme, irrespective of age. They recognise this as being more radical and therefore a greater challenge to existing social security systems. For that reason, however, it would require a major restructuring of public welfare at a time when the broader legitimacy of social welfare as an enterprise is highly contested, although a semi-privatised equitable model of age-related pensions is feasible (Johnson and Falkingham, 1992, p. 187). This partly resembles the situation in Finland, where 42 per cent of 'pensioners' are under 65 years of age, although this system, like others in Scandinavia, is under fiscal pressure (Anttonen, 1991).

To the extent that this new politics of old age is interconnected to the fiscal crises of advanced capitalism it seems likely that it will have an impact also in those countries of Eastern Europe which begin to adapt to more market-orientated economic structures. However, at the same time, the cultural patterns of family relationships and intergenerational expectations in the east resemble those of the south more than the north (Midre and Synak, 1989; Jylhä and Jokela, 1990). Just as there are wide variations of intergenerational expectation between the countries of the EC at present (for example, Greece, Portugal or Spain differ greatly from France, Germany or the UK in this respect), so too the gradual integration of Czechoslovakia, Hungary or Poland into the new Europe will also potentially extend the range of responses to questions of intergenerational equity and citizenship.

It should not be expected that influence through the exchange of ideas between countries will be either deterministic or unidirectional (Jani-Le Bris, 1992). It cannot be expected that whole structures will be copied intact, or that the flow of ideas will be only from the north and west to the south and east. For instance, as Giori (1983) asserts, giving a central role to older people runs contrary to the segregational logic of capitalism, as expressed in the development of pensions or residential homes. So it may be that the influence of those Eastern European countries such as Bulgaria or Romania which appear to have less enthusiasm for a full-scale rush to market mechanisms for health and welfare will find a sympathetic resonance in Scandinavia and some EC countries (such as the UK) where state welfare faces an uncertain future but in which there remains a degree of support towards public provision for needs faced by older people (Minev et al., 1990; Deacon, 1992a; Rose, 1993; Széman and Gáthy, 1993).

The issue of the association between ageing and intergenerational relations has also been identified in the preceding discussion as one of the extent to which families, especially particular members of families, are regarded as having the major responsibility for providing care to older people with dependency needs. There is also an issue as to whether expectations of family obligations are expressed in popular perceptions, contained in formal public policies or incorporated in professional practices.

There may also be differences between what people say they expect and how they actually do act (Finch, 1989). A critical approach to possible future responses to old age in European society cannot ignore this dimension and must recognise the extent to which the role of 'the family' in the lives of older people (as the overwhelming source of informal care as well as of opportunities to make a social contribution) remains a central conceptual and empirical question.

Regional variation and the transfer of ideas

Developments towards a 'new Europe' also extend the range of possibilities in the transfer of specific ideas about policy and practice in the care of older people. The images of Eastern Europe current in the West in the 1990s are dominated by impressions of shortage, poverty and helplessness (Rose, 1993). Concern for children (for instance in Romania) has often been at the centre of Western interest, yet there are positive factors in care for older people which pre-date comparable ideas about good practice in Western European countries. For example, older people have been involved in the practical and decision-making aspects of the management of day-centres and residential homes in Hungary since 1971 (although this has not necessarily countered negative views of institutional care) (Beregi, 1980; Széman and Sik, 1991). This practice, which challenges concepts of the dependent older person as a passive recipient of care, and reinforces citizenship rights, has only more recently begun to be introduced in some EC countries (Clough, 1981; Hunter, 1986; Dieck, 1990; Kraan *et al.*, 1991).

There are also many possibilities for the exchange of ideas between the countries of Western Europe about specific responses to ageing (Fogarty, 1986). Although it may be a rough 'rule of thumb' that the further south one goes in Europe the less well-developed certain services are, yet each country has developed some forms of welfare response that are unique and could stand as illustrations for consideration in other contexts (Jani-Le Bris, 1992; Steenvoorden *et al.*, 1992). Despite the many variations in social structure and relationships that have been discussed at length in previous chapters, there are also sufficient points of similarity to make such a transfer of ideas both possible and potentially fruitful, whether they are about problems being faced or about the success of specific projects or policies. To illustrate this suggestion I want to look in more detail at two such examples, one general and one specific, and then to make some further observations about the utility of an applied comparative approach in considering the development of welfare responses to older people.

Change and Development – Two Examples

Scandinavia: the model of public services

Probably the most highly-developed welfare state structures in Europe have been those of Scandinavia. These countries have had extensive institutional care provision and other supportive services, very high rates of retirement pensions (which have ensured that older people in Scandinavia are well-off relative to other parts of Europe), and there are no legal obligations on families to provide care (Hokenstad and Johansson, 1990; Johansson, 1991; Daatland, 1992). At the same time there has developed widespread ideological support for the use of public services, either as a supplement to or a substitute for family and other informal care (Sundstrøm, 1986; Daatland, 1990; Siim, 1990; Wærness, 1990). As a consequence, the Scandinavian experience has been claimed as a model for other countries attempting to pursue the development of patterns of care which are regarded as appropriate by older people themselves, by their families and within wider society (Little, 1979; Finch, 1984; Ungerson, 1990; Foster, 1991). However, the Scandinavian countries have not, on the one hand, been exempt from the fiscal pressures that have faced other European states, nor on the other hand from the demographic changes that are leading to a marked rise in the proportions of older people, especially those who will require care and support (Anttonen, 1991; Daatland, 1992; Palme and Ståhlborg, 1993). In all Scandinavian countries the proportions of people aged over 80 using such services is very high (averaging 22.75 per cent) and it is in this age group that the highest levels of dependency needs and the largest proportional growth can be seen. In other words, Scandinavia is facing the same immediate future potential demands for care as other European countries (as has been discussed in previous chapters) but on a proportionately slightly larger scale because of its starting point. So to what extent is the Scandinavian system a plausible model for the rest of Europe?

The first question which has to be addressed in considering the applicability of the Scandinavian model of welfare responses to the care needs of older people in other countries is the extent to which it is itself facing rapid change. Changes in the growth in levels of care provision were noted in Sweden in the mid-1980s and by the end of the decade this had become apparent also in Denmark, Finland and Norway (Sundstrøm, 1986; Daatland, 1992). Daatland makes connections between this levelling-off and a concern to control the costs of public spending on services for older people as well as in other areas. The growth in influence of the political New Right, especially in Denmark and Norway, has led to challenges to previously existing consensus assumptions about the proportions of gross national product (GNP) (between 21 and 35 per cent) which are directed to welfare spending, of which older people and their families are the major beneficiaries.

The balance between different types of care services in Scandinavia has also begun to change, with a greater emphasis on community-based provision and an attempt to move away from a heavy reliance on institutions, including a greater use of the latter for respite care or rehabilitation (Daatland, 1992).

In Scandinavia, community care services have developed alongside rather than after institutional care. This can be explained by the late growth of the welfare state (relative to France, Germany or the UK) and by the prevailing form of social democratic relationships between the state and citizens (Siim, 1990; Daatland, 1992). However, there is not an even spread as ten per cent of service users receive half the available number of home care hours (Sundstrøm, 1986; Daatland, 1990). Again, there is a concentration on older elderly people and those people with high levels of dependency needs. In Norway and Sweden there are systems of paid 'family home helpers' through which family carers can be employed by the municipality to undertake a large amount of direct care work for a relative (Wærness, 1990; Johansson, 1991; Kraan *et al.*, 1991). This is intended to recompense informal carers for the loss of employment opportunities which result from the caring role, but unlike comparable measures in other countries (such as the care allowances in Germany or the UK) these schemes constitute employment rather than income support, overcoming any emphasis on an 'unemployed' status for such carers. At the same time it is recognised that this type of employment can only provide part-time employment, is relatively low-paid, and so tends to be directed towards women kin (Wærness, 1990, pp. 124–6; Johansson, 1991, pp. 45–6). Thus it represents a model of advance on other systems in relation to levels and types of remuneration (see the discussion in Chapter 6) while still incorporating some elements of patriarchal values of welfare and caring.

Not only do the form and extent of Scandinavian welfare responses to older people differ from those in other European countries, but also the degree of ideological support for non-family care is much greater, whether this is community- or institution-based, with between 66 and 76 per cent of older people looking to public sources for long-term care (Daatland, 1990, pp. 6–12). Moreover, this expression of choice does not represent a 'rejection' of older people by their families but rather ways of expressing concern (such as by ensuring appropriate services are provided), coupled with a recognition by older people and their families alike of the demands of providing care for a person with increasing frailty (Daatland, 1990, pp. 1–5). The wide use of public services can be seen as a 'retreat from non-reciprocity' in that in those contexts where reciprocity is possible (child-minding by the older person in return for other care received, for example) the social costs of care are often regarded as being more equitably distributed (Sundstrøm, 1986, p. 76).

Increased public emphasis in Scandinavia on care provided directly by the family is part of the creation of the social climate for a wider 'welfare mix', as a means to reduce future projected costs to the state of care provision (Thorslund, 1991). This is in contrast to The Netherlands or the UK, where apparently similar policies have the intention of reducing current levels of public spending, rationing services by using increasingly exclusive definitions of need (Jamieson, 1991c). It is also in contrast to Belgium, France or Germany, where a combination of formal community care is developing alongside emphasis on the family, as a means of stemming the current demands on institutional care, especially in the health sector (Evers and Olk, 1991; Jamieson, 1991c).

In practice, the extent to which intergenerational family solidarity in Scandinavia has remained strong despite changing circumstances can be seen in the adaptation of expectations about who will provide the actual caring work and how this will be provided. For example, in a detailed qualitative study, Johansson (1991, p. 51) recorded the views of older people and their carers that the use of public services as an alternative to family care was often 'reluctantly' seen as 'inevitable', especially when this meant admission to an institutional context. Similarly, Daatland (1990, pp. 6–12) noted that although public services were preferred for long-term care needs, the family was seen as being more appropriate in almost half the instances recorded for short-term care. This was because family care was regarded as being less disruptive. Furthermore, these figures disguise the very large extent to which caring in Scandinavia is already a mixture of public and family provision, with levels of family involvement in the care of older people estimated at between 65 and 75 per cent (Sundstrøm, 1986; Hokenstad and Johansson, 1990). This mixture plays an essential part in the continuation of families providing caring work, as it helps to offset the anxiety felt by some carers that they would be abandoned by the rest of society. It did not, however, prevent some carers experiencing their care work as a 'burden' (Johansson, 1991). What it did mean was that carers were more likely to regard their care work to some extent as a choice and so to find it fulfilling. Where it was not, admissions to residential care were likely to follow, as in other parts of Northern Europe (Thorslund and Johansson, 1987).

In order to examine the transferability of the implications of Scandinavian welfare experience to other European countries, it is necessary to consider two dimensions. These are, first, the types of welfare state which have developed and, second, their connection to wider social relationships and values (especially concerning the family). Daatland (1992) refers to the typology (discussed above) between 'residual', 'insurance' and 'institutional' welfare states. In these terms, and despite the increased fluidity of welfare mixes, the Scandinavian countries are still 'institutional' welfare states, while the remainder of the EC and Eastern Europe can be said to be comprised of either 'residual' or 'insurance' systems. Moreover, in the preceding discussion it has been noted that the direction of change throughout Europe (including Scandinavia) is towards increased reliance on insurance as the basis for access to welfare. For this reason it seems unlikely that the Scandinavian experience of welfare responses to older people can or will provide the model for other European countries without radical and unanticipated changes in economic and political spheres.

At the ideological level it would seem more plausible to think of the Scandinavian experience as a reference point for shifts in social values elsewhere in Europe. In part this is because the high degree of acceptance of public assistance for older people has emerged in response both to the growth in the numbers of older people with dependency needs and to the patterns of women's employment as it affects the availability of family carers (Wærness, 1990). Such changes can be seen in other northern European countries, and in parts of Eastern Europe the legacies of the Communist era include similar patterns (von Ballusek, 1983; Guillemard, 1983; Finch, 1989; Midre and Synak, 1989; Jylhä and Jokela, 1990; Hartl, 1991; Széman, 1992). Yet at the same time the Scandinavian evidence points clearly to a mixture of public and family care, supporting and supplementing families, rather than to the rejection of older people by their families. The idea of a mixed system may provide the basis for a reconsideration of public care services in southern and eastern countries as a means by which family patterns regarding older people can adapt along with other changes, such as women's participation in the labour market. However, as with the structural issues identified above, this will not happen without major public debates and the further politicisation of old age as an issue for general concern.

Greece: the model of open access

Following from the 'rule of thumb' about the north–south spread of services for older people quoted above, there is an underlying notion in many European comparisons that the flow of ideas and practices for the development of welfare responses to old age will be one-way, that is from the north to the south. The previous, more general example of Scandinavia does partly challenge this assumption. The other example I want to consider in this final chapter also questions this presupposition.

The Open Care Centres for Elderly People (KAPI) in Greece, to which brief reference has already been made in preceding chapters, originated in urban Athens in the late 1970s as the result of action in poorer districts by several non-governmental organisations (Dontas, 1987). Following rapid demographic changes in these districts, the initial programmes ended, but the concept was adopted by the government, which in 1981 initiated the wider spread of centres elsewhere in Athens and in other parts of Greece, using municipal funding (Dontas, 1987; Teperoglou *et al.*, 1990). As they are now constituted, the KAPI are staffed by a social worker (usually as director), a nurse, a physiotherapist, an occupational therapist, a home help and a part-time doctor. The centres are accessible to older people who are able to get to them, and provide both a social centre and a point of access to the various professional services that are represented by the staff (as well as through them to other forms of help). Additionally, the centres form a base for home-care provided to those people not able to attend, and for social work in the surrounding area (Teperoglou *et al.*, 1990, p. 20).

In a study of the work of the KAPI and the perceptions of the older people who use them, Teperoglou *et al.* (1990, p. 155) have observed social factors to be the main areas of benefit. Approximately 30 per cent of all elderly people interviewed identified entertainment as the main gain from attendance, and a further 15 per cent distinguished companionship as the principal advantage (see also, Amira, 1990). Only 1 per cent, all of whom were attenders in the Athens area, voiced complaints concerning the sizes and types of building used. This latter point is important to note, however, despite the small proportion complaining, because the KAPI have usually been created in existing premises, which are often older buildings, and this may also affect accessibility. Other criticisms concerned a lack of variety in the programmes and a need for more professional input (Teperoglou *et al.*, 1990, p. 156). One notable suggestion for improvement was in the extent of medical care offered, a point of most concern to women aged over 75 in the areas outside Athens, although only identified by 15 per cent of the respondents.

A significant aspect of the KAPI is that they have open access. In other words, any older person living in an area served by a centre may attend it, and attendance levels can be as high as two-thirds of the eligible population (Dontas, 1987, p. 123). This suggests that the levels of attendance reflect the active choice of the older people concerned, which is reflected in the research findings. Through the centres, therefore, it is possible not only to provide the basic social service of a day centre but also to make the core primary care professionals more freely accessible than would be the case in traditional clinics or hospital settings. For this reason Teperoglou (1990, p. 171) has argued that the KAPI should be developed further.

Some criticisms have been made both of the way in which the KAPI relate to the more general needs faced by older people in Greece and in relation to the impact of the KAPI within the broader welfare framework. First, there is the question of whether the KAPI are able to be used by those who might be in most need. Teperoglou's findings were that on grounds of gender, class, health and age the centres may not have been reaching those older people for whom formal professional assistance might be of most help:

1. The majority of users (55 per cent) are men, although men form a minority of the population aged over 65;
2. The majority of users (between 89 and 96 per cent) had been employed in manual work, although only a minority (17 per cent) did not perceive their financial situation as being average or good;
3. Between 68 and 84 per cent of users reported reasonable health; and
4. The age of attenders was predominantly in the group under 75 years of age (between 67.5 and 78.6 per cent) (Teperoglou *et al.* 1990, p. 30, pp. 43–4, pp. 87–8).

Not only are the KAPI, therefore, not necessarily reaching the older people who are most in need of access to professional care, but they have been described by Dontas (1987, p. 126) as being expensive. This high relative cost is set against the alternative model of experimental geriatric clinics in local health centres, which have been abandoned in the course of developing the national health services.

However, Dontas does not address the question of open access: he concentrates on the question of delivering help to those who are in immediate need, and we are returned to the issue of needs against rights, the rationing and targeting of services, and the questions of citizenship and social access. It may be that in promoting the self-determination of older people to make use of services they value that those who are most at risk, particularly in relation to their health, are served less well. The outworking from the KAPI described by Teperoglou *et al.* (19992) might be one solution to this, but the limitations of resources have also been identified. It would appear that open access has the potential to be a useful device for putting older people in contact with professional help before they need to make use of it, but such a preventative focus is not highly developed at present.

Furthermore, Dontas (1987, p. 123) is critical that the KAPI have had an unintended impact on the cultural situation of older Greeks. Of special note in the Greek context is the way in which it encourages a mixing of the sexes, which was not culturally normative among older Greeks, but segregates different age groups in the process compared to the more traditional meeting-places of coffee-house and doorstep. In this sense it could be observed that the pattern of social relationships developing through the KAPI more closely resembles that of northern Europe and might bring with it the parallel problem of the separation of the generations. In recent years some gerontologists and older people themselves have begun to argue that mutuality will not emerge from, but be stifled through, segregation of this kind (Hagestad, 1986; Kuhn, 1986). Not only may the ordinary opportunities for intergenerational contact diminish but there is a related problem of possible stigmatisation which in other countries has accompanied service segregation. However, there is no evidence of this in Greece at the present time.

The ideas contained within the development of the KAPI can be seen elsewhere in Europe, for example in Portugal, where open access day centres for older people have also existed since the late 1970s and are becoming more available, or in Scandinavia where the principles of KAPI are replicated and in some instances the concept has been borrowed explicitly from Greece (Olsen, 1991; Steenvoorden *et al.*, 1992; Daatland, 1992). In the latter examples, however, there is a much more deliberate attempt to create services to support family carers through the provision of domestic support as well as day-care, and less emphasis on preventative health work. For example, the Portuguese model has a number of home helps who work out from the centre, which in effect forms a community base in addition to drawing the community into the centre. The German development of *Sozialstationen*, in contrast, were established in the 1970s with similar objectives, but have tended to become bases for professionals providing care in older people's own homes rather than functioning as centres to which older people can go for psychosocial support (Evers and Olk, 1991).

Both the Greek and the Portuguese approaches to day-care have much to offer areas of northern Europe, where the more institutional focus has tended to produce professionally-orientated day-care, without open access, which is separated from the surrounding community. This promotion of self-determination among older people is a factor which distinguishes the southern European model, even though there is less of a focus on direct health care. Moreover, a study in the UK, showed that attenders at sampled day-care centres spent only approximately 30 per cent of their time in contact with other people, and that most did not have anything to do for much of the time (Godlove *et al.*, 1982). The hub of the work of the KAPI is in providing communal activities for the centres' members, and this was a highly valued part of the service. In this regard it would seem that the Mediterranean model, especially that which has been developed in Greece, could serve as an illustration for more northern European countries.

General issues of transferability

Throughout this book I have stressed the extent to which it is important to consider the differences as well as the similarities between national contexts, and the illustrative examples of Scandinavia and Greece are sketched out on that basis. Each specific situation is based in the overall patterns of care for older people and the position they occupy more generally in society. For that reason it is not suggested that any particular model or set of issues is directly transferable to another context without some critical thought. What is intended to be shown in these two illustrations is the ways in which local concerns have wider implications. First, the rapid pace of change may present the most highly developed pattern of care for older people with a challenge, not only of direction but possibly also to the core ideologies. It may be that the questioning of the state basis of care for older people in Scandinavia marks the potential limit of that direction of development across the whole of Europe, at least in the foreseeable future. Second, even in these circumstances it remains a positive step to consider an interchange of ideas containing elements of mutuality, ordinary life and self-determination rather than assumptions about a general movement towards the institutionalising of care for elderly people in state agencies. The KAPI of Greece serve as just such an illustration, which is a useful starting point in spite of the problems identified above, precisely because it has emerged from a context in which there was little alternative and a growing need for new provision (Teperoglou *et al.*, 1990, p. 171).

Each European country has some development of services to older people, or their families, which might provide a basis for review and further development in another national context (Jamieson, 1991c; Steenvoorden *et al.*, 1992). What is needed to enable this to take place on wider scale is a recognition of the commonalities and the differences between the needs of older people in the various countries and a comparative perspective on the social structures and relationships of which they are a part. The adaptation of the KAPI to Scandinavia provides just one example of how this might be considered in a way which goes beyond a stereotype of the spread of the 'institutional' view of the state (in Titmuss's terms) from the north to the south. The emergence of the new Europe may enable this interchange to take place more effectively. Certainly, it is occurring at a time when a search for new ideas and practices is becoming increasingly necessary, and the idea of a welfare mix is becoming increasingly widespread.

An Older European Society

European trends

Two broad trends can be discerned in the preceding discussion. The first reflects a concern with the growing scale of needs among older people, arising from the demographic changes which throughout but the 1980s have come to be labelled 'the ageing society' (de Jouvenal, 1988); the second is an interest in promoting old age as a valued part of the life-cycle, in challenging the 'crisis of identity' with a more positive perception (Kuhn, 1986).

To the extent that the important question for policy-makers and professionals has become that of sustaining welfare responses to need in old age in a context of potentially growing demand, discussions about ageing will be dominated by a new concept of older people as a social 'burden'. This is indeed what has happened, with the idea of the 'age war' (Estes, 1986), and is a key concern in the development of new welfare mixes (Svetlik, 1991). The potential outcome is that in order to resolve the conflict of interests inherent in this situation, the social categorisation of older people into those who are 'deserving' and those who are 'undeserving' which informed the early days of institutional care will be revived within European old-age policies (Gruman, 1978). The recent changes in Scandinavia discussed earlier contain the seeds of such a change, which can be seen also in the UK and other Northern countries (Walker, 1990; Daatland, 1992).

In contrast to the perceived difference between older and younger people, the potential of community care has been seized as an opportunity for a welfare response which is based on ordinariness, and so can be regarded positively by older people themselves as well as by critics of institutions. Moreover, some of the support for community-based services has derived from the perception that they are a cheap alternative. However, detailed analysis of experimental schemes in the UK has shown that although the monthly unit cost per person may be lower, the overall costs are likely to be higher if people live longer as a result of the care they receive (Chesterman *et al.*, 1988). This difference arises from the increased use of acute medical services by older people who remain in the community, and the costs of housing subsidy. It may represent cost-effectiveness, in the sense of the relationship between cost and quality, but it is difficult to sustain an argument about reduced costs if these are regarded in total.

The other dimension to the emphasis on community or home-based care is in the implications for family carers. As the feminist critics in particular have noted, costing community care in monetary terms does not account for the social costs of effort by family members who are usually spouses or women of the immediately younger generation (Green, 1988; Hicks, 1988). The point, discussed earlier, is that in all European countries much care for older people is provided already within or by the family. The concern at a European level, for example within the EC, about the impact of 'the ageing society' on carers can be seen, therefore, as part of the overall direction in policy towards creating and sustaining the conditions in which increasing numbers of older people with dependency needs can continue to live in the community without a matching increase in the levels of public provision (Council of Europe, 1991b; Jani-Le Bris, 1992). Support for carers can be seen to be emerging, even in countries where previously the family was simply assumed to be the natural base of caring (Anderson, 1992).

It is at this juncture that the potential for conflict of interest between older people and the younger members of their families may arise. Community services and home-based care may be the desired alternatives because they enhance positive images of older people through being located in ordinary social surroundings. However, as we noted, it may do so at the cost of demands placed on family carers which conflict with their capacity to engage in ordinary social life. It is possible as a consequence that Europe is moving towards a situation in which the contradictions contained within community-care policies will be increasingly heightened.

This point is illustrated in the following hypothetical example. If I wish to remain in my own home but I require assistance because of disabilities which have increased as I have grown older, in all European countries my first source of help will be my family. If both I and they find this acceptable then there is no conflict. However, conflict can arise for several reasons, because it disrupts the family life of my younger relatives or because the direct costs in giving up work (despite carers' allowances or 'employment' as a carer) may be greater than they are able to bear. In such a case there will be a limit to the extent of community care available, and it is likely that I will be faced with admission to residential care, not as a choice but as a necessity. As has already been discussed above, even in those countries where residential care is relatively well accepted there is still an ethos of 'having to' rather than 'choosing to' (Foster, 1991; Johansson, 1991; Széman and Sik, 1991; Allen *et al.*, 1992). In such a context the psychological and social costs that have to be borne by both the older person and the family carers are considerable.

This dilemma, of resolving the potential differences between the interests of older people and their family carers can be seen predominantly as one of equality of opportunity and social access. The impact of the overall direction in European social policy development appears at one level to be to privatise any conflict within the family (Dieck, 1987 and 1990). However, this seems likely to make more explicit the social as well as the economic costs involved in creating a full range of alternatives for care of older people. At another level this is offset by the goals of using formal services to supplement informal care, in the welfare mix. Yet the actual volume and coverage of services will be vital, because without a sufficient level of provision the sense of potential conflict will not be resolved, as the rationing and targeting inherent in these approaches will highlight the contested nature of need. It will not be possible to avoid recognising that the choices which are made reflect perspectives taken on the ageing enterprise as a whole, and not just a minority of 'elderly people' from whom the majority can remain discrete.

In Chapter 4, reference was made to the social-anthropological evidence of 'geronticide', that is, the deliberate killing of older people constituted as a 'burden' in some pre-industrial societies (de Beauvoir, 1977). It was noted also that the 'age war' arguments which 'favour' younger people ultimately lead to a metaphorical 'social geronticide', and at the extreme to literal manifestations through the withholding of medical treatments (de Jouvenal, 1988, p. 47). Clearly, this is not a scientific choice but one of ethics and politics. The images of old age which are constructed through welfare responses to dependency needs (including pensions, transport and housing as well as health and social-care services) are intrinsically bound up with the images of European society as a whole. Ageism is not just to be found in media and advertising portrayals of older people, or in colloquialisms and jokes (although these are powerful carriers of cultural messages) but is endemic in the economic, political and cultural assumptions which inform the development and operation of the major European social institutions, the professions and wider community life.

An important aspect of this growing crisis in the identity of old age has been the past construction of older people as passive recipients rather than as active participants in the enterprise (Elder, 1977; Guillemard, 1983; Bornat *et al.*, 1985; Fogarty, 1986; Hagestad, 1986; Dieck, 1987). It is for this reason I would suggest that one of the key implications from the example of the KAPI in Greece (see above) should be seen as their open access. This emphasises the active role of the older person in making choices about whether to attend, when to attend and so on. I recognise that such choices, like any which we make, do not occur in a situation of absolute discretion: the interests of other family members or the range of possible alternatives, for example, may play a part in the decision which is reached. Nevertheless, the general point remains that in an open access model the older person is an active participant in all aspects of the caring service, including the initial decision, rather than just a passive recipient.

Two alternative perspectives have been developed to counter the one-dimensional view of old age as being passive. The first is to consider the contribution made by older people to contemporary society, while the second is to concentrate on the ordinary citizenship of older people in a context where quite specific social roles are allocated (for example, being no longer eligible for paid employment, as discussed in Chapter 3).

Older people may be regarded as being contributors to contemporary society in two ways: both through their previous work in paid employment and in domestic labour, or in their current activities. The concept of past contribution to the present is an idea which could exercise a powerful influence, employing the logic that current care in some way represents a repayment of a debt for past labour, a use of accumulated 'social capital'. However, the anti-welfarist ideology which now prevails across Europe denies this through its emphasis on private monetary capital as the basis for access to all areas of social life. For this reason, strategies for enhancing the cultural identity of older people based on the idea of past contribution seem relatively weak.

The recognition of the current contribution of older people to contemporary society is therefore a much stronger concept. In both the home and the community older people make large, but often unacknowledged, contributions to society. One example of this is in the performing of domestic labour or in undertaking child-care (Allen *et al.*, 1992; Hörl, 1992; Stathopoulos and Amera, 1992). The prevailing tendency in Europe against co-residence does not prevent reciprocal care from being a widespread reality, particularly among family members (Pitsiou, 1986; Finch, 1989; Pijl, 1991).

Outside the family, older people also make a hidden social contribution, often through voluntary work of various kinds, including both the control of services for themselves and the provision of care to other older people who have different needs or greater levels of dependency. This point is identified in an EC study which quotes details of a wide range of associations and social clubs in Belgium, France, Germany and The Netherlands, as well as social welfare provision being delivered by older people to other older people in the Irish Republic, Germany and the UK (Fogarty, 1986). Dieck (1990, p. 115) describes the German self-help scene in particular as being 'vivacious' and 'active'. Examples include the delivery of meals-on-wheels, shopping, visiting schemes and counselling. Moreover, such reciprocity is not confined to groups of older people (which may in itself be intergenerational) but encompasses younger people with dependency needs and other forms of service within the locality. A major resource which older people tend to have is time, and Fogarty's study concluded that this would be a positive policy to build on, and to incorporate the active potential of older people (Fogarty, 1986, p. 95). At the same time it noted that traditions of giving voluntary service might have both a national and a class dimension, and there may need to be more organised encouragement and support for older people to make this type of response. However, the very same older people's associations could provide the basis for this to happen.

Active participation of older people in European society within a privatised conception of needs and interests, for example as a wealthy consumer, is divisive to the extent that different groups of older people do not have access to the means to enable them to participate. This is particularly so when the model of activity differs from that of passivity only in so far as it involves the power of choice derived from control over economic resources. Attempts to find commonalities in the active contribution of older people in direct forms (for example, in voluntary service which may be for the benefit of younger people as well as other older people) in this way challenges the inherent ageism which characterises old age as a time only of inactivity and consumption.

Towards a Europe for older people

Analysis and action in the 'ageing society' of Europe has been dominated by policy-makers and professionals, although there are some notable exceptions (Elder, 1977). In recent years there has been a growing emphasis within such work on the importance of understanding the variety of circumstances and experiences which constitutes older age (Walker, 1986b; Fennell *et al.*, 1988). Such an understanding is vital to correct the monolithic view of 'old age' which failed to take into account differences in class, gender, race, ethnicity, disability or even age itself, as was discussed in previous chapters. This is a reflection of the exclusion of older people, or at least certain older people, from public life, as well as other social divisions within the professions, the scientific community and government.

At the same time, paradoxically, the monolithic view of ageing sustains a lack of identity among older people as members of the wider society with interests in common with others age groups (Walker, 1986b). This might include the benefits to all members of society in developing or sustaining public health and welfare – provision, to family carers as well as directly to older people. It would also include attempts to counter ageism in European culture and popular thought. The model in the USA has been that of the Gray Panthers, which differs from older people's associations in Europe in the extent to which it has sought to politicise old age, while at the same time stressing the extent to which the interests of older people are congruent with the interests of all groups within society (Kuhn, 1986; Dieck, 1987 and 1990). This is not only in the sense of saying that the individual members of current younger generations have an increased likelihood of growing old, than its members of previous generations although it does include that fact, but also that for the most part the struggles of older people have great similarity to struggles among other age groups at the present time. For example, services that are paternalistic and demeaning should be challenged on that basis rather than because one specific age group does not find this acceptable. So the Gray Panthers include in their membership not only those people who might be defined as 'old' (ignoring the practical and theoretical problems of such a definition) but also of anyone else who wishes to engage with this cause.

Commentators on the European context have not detected a comparable politicisation of old age in the sense of an intergenerational multi-issue organisation. In the UK Phillipson (1982) identifies a 'vertical fragmentation' of political action even in relation to issues such as pensions. In part this is a consequence of psychological ageism: 'older people are other and not me'. Much of the argument is then left up to older people themselves. In the UK the National Council of Older People has joined with trade unions to mount campaigns, while in Sweden, pensioners' organisations are the main protagonists against reductions in formal welfare provision (Bornat *et al.*, 1985; Kraan *et al.*, 1991). In Germany municipal authorities have supported the creation of representative 'councils of elderly people', but these tend to work as lobbyists within the existing structures and only a minority of older Germans are involved (Dieck, 1990). However, for the most part, younger people tend not to be involved. The negative images associated with ageing are integral to the lack of will to contest reductions in pension levels or health and welfare provision, because, as these have existed in Europe, they have been founded in effect on a social contract between generations.

For Europe to become an 'ageing society' in the fullest sense of the word: that is, a society *for* as well as *of* older people, it will be necessary for images of old age as well for institutional responses to be developed positively. As was shown in the earlier part of this book, Europe, in relation to old age as well as in other aspects, is not a monolith, but contains a diversity of cultural forms. The risk for southern countries in losing such positive aspects of the social role of older people in the family as remain, through the process of gaining more widely available formal welfare provision, is one which should be considered with some caution. Although such changes may follow from structural developments in the economy, a greater awareness on the part of professionals and policy-makers of the positive contribution by older people to their society will be an important dimension to future practice and planning.

Given the patterns of increased dependence associated with increased ageing it would appear to be crucial also that positive images of old age are promoted even when this involves the provision of health and welfare services. The separation of different groups of older people on the grounds of their varying circumstances, as observed above, could lead potentially to the further demarcation of 'old ages': some positive, others negative. This would not represent an end to ageism but rather a new variation. For this reason, although the discovery of older travellers exploring new horizons may redress a welfarist image, by the same token the reality for a proportion of older people, which increases with advancing age, is one of need for various forms of assistance with daily life (see Chapter 4). Can a positive image be promoted for that part of ageing which may be about need rather than about fun? The answer must depend on the extent to which particular images of old age, based on a concern about welfare needs, exclude others. There is not necessarily a mutual opposition between an older person using intensive domiciliary care and having a fulfilling and positive life, including loving relationships, an opportunity to make a contribution to the lives of others and, indeed, having fun. Where someone does have a need for intensive assistance, the objective should be one of enabling that person to take part in society to the fullest possible extent, and of promoting equality of access and opportunity. This is the challenge created by the ageing of Europe, and it is one which necessarily intertwines the ageing enterprise as a whole and care for those older people who are in need.

Bibliography

ABRAHAMSON, P. (1991) 'Welfare for the Elderly in Denmark: From Institutionalization to Self-reliance', in A. Evers and I. Svetlik (eds), *New Welfare Mixes in Care for the Elderly* (vol. 2) (Vienna: European Centre for Social Welfare Policy and Research).

ABRAMS, P. (1978) *Beyond Three Score and Ten* (London: Age Concern).

ACHENBAUM, W. A. and P. N. STEARNS (1978) 'Old Age and Modernization', *The Gerontologist*, 18 (3), pp. 307–12.

ALLEN, I., D. HOGG and S. PEACE (1992) *Elderly People: Choice, Participation and Satisfaction* (London: Policy Studies Institute).

AMANN, A. (1980a) 'Open Care for the Elderly – Austria', in A. Amann (ed.), *Open Care for the Elderly in Seven European Countries* (Oxford: Pergamon Press).

AMANN, A. (1980b) 'Older People and the Care System – A General Discussion', in A. Amann (ed.), *Open Care for the Elderly in Seven European Countries* (Oxford: Pergamon Press).

AMIRA, A. (1990) 'Family Care in Greece', in A. Jamieson and R. Illsley (eds), *Contrasting European Policies for the Care of Older People* (Aldershot: Avebury).

ANDERSON, M. (1971) 'Family, Household and the Industrial Revolution', in M. Anderson (ed.), *The Family* (Harmondsworth: Penguin).

ANDERSON, M. (1977) 'The Impact on the Family Relationships of the Elderly of Changes since Victorian Times in Governmental Income-maintenance Provision', in E. Shanas and M. B. Sussman (eds), *Family Bureaucracy and the Elderly* (Durham, N. C.: Duke University Press).

ANDERSON, R. (1992) 'Health and Community Care', in L. Davies (ed.), *The Coming of Age in Europe* (London: Age Concern).

ANDERSSON, L. (1992) 'Family Care of the Elderly in Sweden', in I. J. Kosberg (ed.), *Family Care of the Elderly* (Newbury Park: Sage).

ANTTONEN, A. (1991) 'Care for the Elderly in Finland and the Future of the Scandinavian Caring State', in A. Evers and I. Svetlik (eds), *New Welfare Mixes in Care for the Elderly* (vol. 2) (Vienna: European Centre for Social Welfare Policy and Research).

ANWAR, M. (1979) *The Myth of Return* (London: Heinemann).

ARBER, S. and N. GILBERT (1989) 'Men: The Forgotten Carers', *Sociology*, 23 (1), pp. 111–18.

ARBER, S. and J. GINN (1991) *Gender and Later Life*, (London: Sage).

ASAD, T. (1973) 'Two European Images of Non-European Rule', in T. Asad (ed.), *Anthropology and the Colonial Encounter* (London: Ithaca Press).

BALLUSEK, H. von (1983) 'Origins and Trends of Social Policy for the Aged in the Federal Republic of Germany and West Berlin', in A.-M. Guillemard (ed.), *Old Age and the Welfare State* (London: Sage).

174

BANK-MIKKELSON, N. (1976) 'Denmark', in R. Kugel and A. Shearer (eds), *Changing Patterns of Residential Services for the Mentally Handicapped* (revised edition) (Washington, D.C.: President's Committee for the Mentally Retarded).

BARKER, J. (1984) *Black and Asian Old People in Britain* (Mitcham: Age Concern).

BARNES, J. (1979) *Who Should Know What?* (Harmondsworth: Penguin).

BARO, F., L. MOORTHAMER, G. de BRUYNE, H. VAN DEN BERG, and K. MAGITS (1991) 'Home-care Services in the Flanders, Belgium', in A. Jamieson (ed.), *Home Care for Older People in Europe* (Oxford University Press).

BEAUVOIR, S. de (1977) (trans. P. O'Brian) *Old Age* (Harmondsworth: Penguin).

BECKER, H. S. (1967) 'Whose Side Are We On?', *Social Problems*, 14 (3), pp. 239–47.

BELL, D. (1973) *The Coming of Post-Industrial Society* (New York: Harper & Row).

BENDIX, R. (1966) *Max Weber: An Intellectual Portrait* (London: Methuen and Co).

BEREGI, E. (1980) 'Hungary', in E. Palmore (ed.), *International Handbook on Ageing: Contemporary Developments and Research* (London: Macmillan).

BERGER, P. (1979) *Facing up to Modernity* (Harmondsworth: Penguin).

BEVERFELT, E. (1980) 'Norway', in E. Palmore (ed.), *International Handbook on Ageing: Contemporary Developments and Research* (London: Macmillan).

BHALLA, A. and K. BLAKEMORE (1981) *Elderly of the Ethnic Minority Groups* (Birmingham: All Faiths for One Race).

BIANCHI, M. (1991) 'Policy for the Elderly in Italy: Innovation or Modernization?', in A. Evers and I. Svetlik (eds), *New Welfare Mixes in Care for the Elderly* (vol. 3) (Vienna: European Centre for Social Welfare Policy and Research).

BIGGS, S. (1989) 'Professional Helpers and Resistances to Work with Older People', *Ageing and Society*, 9 (1), pp. 43–60.

BINNEY, E. A. and C. ESTES (1988) 'The Retreat of the State and its Transformed Response: The Intergenerational War', *International Journal of Health Services*, 18 (1), pp. 83–96.

BLAKELY, B. E. and R. DOLON (1991) 'The Relative Contributions of Occupation Groups in the Discovery and Treatment of Elder Abuse and Neglect', *Journal of Gerontological Social Work*, 17 (1/2), pp. 183–99.

BLAKEMORE, K. (1985) 'The State, the Voluntary Sector and New Developments in Provision for the Old of Minority Racial Groups', *Ageing and Society*, 5 (2), pp. 175–90.

BLOMMERSTIJN, P. (1980) 'Open Care for the Elderly – The Netherlands', in A. Amann (ed.), *Open Care for the Elderly in Seven European Countries* (Oxford: Pergamon Press).

BLYTHE, R. (1972) *Akenfield: Portrait of an English Village* (Harmondsworth: Penguin).

BOERI, T. (1993) 'Unemployment in Central and Eastern Europe: Transient or Persistent?', in S. Ringen and C. Wallace (eds), *Societies in Transition: East-Central Europe Today* (Prague: Central European University).

BONANUS, A. and T. M. CALASANTI (1986) 'The Status of Rural Elderly in Southern Italy', *Ageing and Society*, 6 (1), pp. 13–37.

BOND, J. (1986) 'Political Economy as a Perspective in the Analysis of Old Age', in C. Phillipson, M. Bernard and P. Strang (eds), *Dependency and Interdependency in Old Age – Theoretical Perspectives and Policy Alternatives* (London: Croom Helm).

BOND, J. (1990) 'Living Arrangements of Elderly People', in J. Bond and P. Coleman (eds), *Ageing in Society* (London: Sage).

BOND, J., R. BRIGGS and P. COLEMAN (1990) 'The Study of Ageing', in J. Bond and P. Coleman (eds), *Ageing in Society* (London: Sage).

BOOTH, C. (1892) *Pauperism and the Endowment of Old Age* (London: Macmillan).

BOOTH, T. (1985) *Home Truths: Old People's Homes and the Outcome of Care* (Aldershot: Gower).

BORNAT, J., C. PHILLIPSON and S. WARD (1985) *A Manifesto for Old Age* (London: Pluto Press).

BRADSHAW, J. (1972) 'The Concept of Social Need', *New Society*, 19, pp. 640–3.

BRAVERMAN, H. (1974) *Labor and Monopoly Capital* (New York: Monthly Review Press).

BREARLEY, C. P. (1975) *Social Work, Ageing and Society* (London: Routledge & Kegan Paul).

BREARLEY, C. P. (1978) 'Ageing and Social Work', in D. Hobman (ed.), *The Social Challenge of Ageing* (London: Croom Helm).

BRECKMAN, S. R. and R. D. ADELMAN (1988) *Strategies for Helping Victims of Elder Mistreatment* (Beverly Hills, Calif.: Sage).

BRIGGS, A. (1968) *Victorian Cities* (Harmondsworth: Penguin).

BRIGGS, R. (1990) 'Biological Ageing', in J. Bond and P. Coleman (eds), *Ageing in Society* (London: Sage).

BRITTAN, A. and M. MAYNARD (1984) *Sexism, Racism and Oppression* (Oxford: Basil Blackwell).

BROCKLEHURST, J. (1978) 'Ageing and Health', in D. Hobman (ed.), *The Social Challenge of Ageing* (London: Croom Helm).

BROWNE, M. (1990) 'Innovation and Linkage in Service Provision for Elderly People in Ireland', in A. Jamieson and R. Illsley (eds), *Contrasting European Policies for the Care of Older People* (Aldershot: Avebury).

BRYAN, D., S. DADZIE and S. SCAFE (1985) *The Heart of the Race* (London: Virago).

BULMER, M. (1987) *The Social Basis of Community Care* (London: George Allen & Unwin).

BURROW, J. A. (1986) *The Ages of Man: A Study in Mediaeval Writing and Thought* (Oxford: Clarendon Press).

BYTHEWAY, W. R. (1980) 'United Kingdom', in E. Palmore (ed.), *International Handbook on Ageing: Contemporary Developments and Research* (London: Macmillan).

CALLAHAN, D. (1986) 'Adequate Health Care and an Ageing Society', *Daedalus*, 115, pp. 247–67.

CALLAHAN, J. J. (1988) 'Elder Abuse: Some Questions for Policy Makers', *The Gerontologist*, 28 (4), pp. 453–8.

CAMERON, E., H. EVERS, F. BADGER and K. ATKIN (1989) 'Black Old Women and Health Carers', in M. Jeffreys (ed.), *Growing Old in the Twentieth Century* (London: Routledge & Kegan Paul).

CAMPOS, A. C. de (1980) *Population Institutionalisée dans le Department de Lisbonne* (Lisbon: École Nationale de Santé Publique).

CARROLL, B. (1991) 'Care for elderly people in Ireland', *Social Policy and Administration*, 25 (3), pp. 238–48.

CASTLE-KANEROVA, M. (1992) 'Social Policy in Czechoslovakia', in B. Deacon (ed.), *The New Eastern Europe* (London: Sage).

CHANDLER, J. T., J. R. RACHAL and R. KAZELSKIS (1986) 'Attitudes of Long-term Care Nursing Personnel toward the Elderly', *The Gerontologist*, 26 (5), pp. 551–5.

CHALLIS, D. 'Case Management: Problems and Possibilities', in I. Allen (ed.) (1990) *Care Managers and Care Management* (London: Policy Studies Institute).

CHALLIS, D. and B. DAVIES (1986) *Case Management in Community Care* (Aldershot: Gower).

CHALLIS, D., R. CHESSUM, J. CHESTERMAN, R. LUCKETT and B. WOODS (1988) 'Community Care for the Frail Elderly: An Urban Experiment', *British Journal of Social Work*, 18 (supplement), pp. 13–42.

CHAUVIRÉ, Y. (1987) 'La géographie des ménages âgés en France et son évolution de 1962 à 1982', in D. Nion and A. Warnes (eds), *Personnes Agées et Vieillissment* (Lille: Espaces-Populations-Sociétés).

CHESTERMAN, J., D. CHALLIS and B. DAVIES (1988) 'Long-term Care at Home for the Elderly: A Four-year Follow-up', *British Journal of Social Work*, 18 (supplement), pp. 43–54.

CLEIRPPA (Centre de Liaison, d'Étude, d'Information et de Recherche sur les Problèmes des Personnes Agées) (1990) *Accueillir Chez Soi une Personne Agées* (Bergerac: La SNEPIA).

CLOGG, R. (1976) *The Movement for Greek Independence 1770–1821* (London: Macmillan).

CLOGG, R. (1986) *A Short History of Modern Greece* (2nd edn) (Cambridge University Press).

CLOUGH, R. (1981) *Old Age Homes*(London: George Allen & Unwin).

COLEMAN, P. and J. BOND (1990) 'Ageing in the Twentieth Century', in J. Bond and P. Coleman (eds), *Ageing in Society* (London: Sage).

COLLINS, J. (1989) *Survey of a Geriatric Day Hospital*, unpublished M.Sc. thesis (Manchester: University of Manchester).

Council of Europe (1991a) *European Co-operation on Social and Family Policy*, RS-INF (91) 1 (Strasbourg: Council of Europe).

Council of Europe (1991b) *Varieties of Welfare Provision and Dependent Old People*, PS-PAF (91) 12 (Strasbourg: Council of Europe).

Council of Europe (1992) *Violence Against Elderly People* (Strasbourg: Council of Europe Press).

COVEY, H. C. (1989) 'Perceptions and Attitudes toward Sexuality of the Elderly during the Middle Ages', *The Gerontologist*, 29 (1), pp. 93–100.

COVEY, H. C. (1991) 'Old Age and Historical Examples of the Miser', *The Gerontologist*, 31 (5), pp. 673–8.

COWGILL, D. O. (1972) 'A Theory of Aging in Cross-cultural Perspective', in D. O. Cowgill and L. D. Holmes (eds), *Aging and Modernization* (New York: Appleton–Century–Crofts).

COWGILL, D. O. and L. D. HOLMES (1972) 'Summary and Conclusions: The Theory in Review', in D. O. Cowgill and L. D. Holmes (eds), *Aging and Modernization* (New York: Appleton–Century–Crofts).

CUMMING, E. and W. E. HENRY (1961) *Growing Old* (New York: Basic Books).

DAATLAND, S. O. (1983) 'Care systems', *Ageing and Society*, 3 (1), pp. 1–21.
DAATLAND, S. O. (1990) 'What Are Families For?', *Ageing and Society*, 10 (1), pp. 1–15.
DAATLAND, S. O. (1992) 'Ideals Cost? Current Trends in Scandinavian Welfare Policy on Ageing', in *Journal of European Social Policy*, 2 (1), pp. 33–47.
DALLEY, G. (1988) *Ideologies of Caring: Rethinking Community and Collectivism* (London: Macmillan).
DAUNT P., (1992) 'Transport and mobility – a European overview', in L. Davies (ed.), *The Coming of Age in Europe* (London: Age Concern).
DAVIES, B. and S. MISSIAKOULIS (1988) 'Heineken and Matching Processes in the Thanet Community Care Project: An Empirical Test of their Relative Importance', *British Journal of Social Work*, 18 (supplement), pp. 55–78.
DAVIS, A. (1981) *The Residential Solution* (London: Tavistock).
DAVIS, L. (1982) *Residential Care: A Community Resource* (London: Heinemann).
DEACON, B. (1992a) 'East European Welfare: Past, Present and Future in Comparative Context', in B. Deacon (ed.), *The New Eastern Europe* (London: Sage).
DEACON, B. (1992b) 'Social Welfare Developments in Eastern Europe and the Future for Socialist Welfare', in P. Carter, T. Jeffs and M. K. Smith (eds), *Changing Social Work and Welfare* (Buckingham: Open University Press).
DHSS (Department of Health and Social Security) (1982) *Growing Older*, Cmnd. 8173 (London: HMSO).
DIECK, M. (1987) 'Gewalt gegen ältere Menschen im familialen Kontext – ein Thema der Forschung, der Praxis und der öffentlich Information', *Zeitschrift für Gerontologie*, 20 (5), pp. 305–13.
DIECK, M. (1990) 'Politics for elderly people in the FDR', in A. Jamieson and R. Illsley (eds), *Contrasting European Policies for the Care of Older People* (Aldershot: Avebury).
DIECK, M. and G. Naegele (1989) 'Die "neuen Älten" – Soziale Ungleichheiten vertiefen sich', in F. Karl and W.Tokarski (eds), *Die 'Neuen' Älten* (Kassel: Gesamthochshulbibliotek).
Dirección General de Juventud y Promoción Socio-cultural (1981) *Acción Cultural con Adultos el Aula de Tercera Edad* (Madrid: Ministerio de Cultura).
DITTMAN-KOHLI, F. (1990) 'The construction of meaning in old age', *Ageing and Society*, 10 (3), pp. 279–94.
DOBASH, R. E. and R. P. DOBASH (1992) *Women, Violence and Social Change* (London: Routledge & Kegan Paul)
DOH (Department of Health) (1989) *Caring for People*, Cm. 849 (London: HMSO).
DOH (Department of Health) (1990) *National Health Service and Community Care Act* (London: HMSO).
DONOVAN, J. (1986) *We Don't Buy Sickness It Just Comes* (Aldershot: Gower).
DONTAS, A. S. (1987) 'Primary Social and Health Services for the Aged in Greece', in S. di Gregorio *Social Gerontology: New Directions* (London: Croom Helm).
DONTAS, A. S., J. H. TRIANTAFILLOU and E. MESTHENEOS (1991) *Policy and Services for the Elderly in Greece* (unpublished report) (Athens: Center of Studies of Age-Related Changes in Man).
DRURY, E. (1992) 'Employment and retirement in Europe', in L. Davies (ed.), *The Coming of Age in Europe* (London: Age Concern).

EASTMAN, M. (1984) *Old Age Abuse* (London: Age Concern).

EHRENREICH, B. and D. ENGLISH (1979) *For Her Own Good* (London: Pluto Press).

ELDER, G. (1977) *The Alienated: Growing Older Today* (London: Writers' and Readers' Co-operative).

ELDRIDGE, J. E. T. (1971) *Max Weber: the Interpretation of Social Reality* (London: Michael Joseph).

ESPING-ANDERSEN, G. (1990) *The Three Worlds of Welfare Capitalism* (Cambridge: Polity Press).

ESTES, C. (1979) *The Aging Enterprise* (San Francisco: Jossey-Bass).

ESTES, C. (1986) 'The Aging Enterprise: In Whose Interests?', *International Journal of Health Services*, 16 (2), pp. 243–51.

EUROLINK AGE (1992) 'The grey agenda', *Eurolink Age Bulletin* (July) (pp. 1–3) (London: Age Concern).

EUROSTAT (1990) *Inequality and Poverty in Europe* (Luxembourg: Office for Official Publications of the European Community).

EUROSTAT (1991) *Demographic Statistics 1991* (Luxembourg: Office for Official Publications of the European Community).

EVANDROU, M. (1992) *Challenging the Invisibility of Carers* in F. Laziko and C. Victor (eds) *Social Policy and Older People* (Aldershot: Gower).

EVANDROU, M., S. ARBER, A. DALE and G. N. GILBERT (1986) 'Who cares for the elderly?', in C. Phillipson, M. Bernard and P. Strang (eds), *Dependency and Interdependency in Old Age – Theoretical Perspectives and Policy Alternatives* (London: Croom Helm).

EVERS, A. and H. WINTERSBERGER (eds) (1988) *Shifts in the Welfare Mix* (Frankfurt: Campus Verlag).

EVERS, A. and T. OLK (1991) 'The Mix of Care Provisions for the Frail Elderly in the Federal Republic of Germany', in A. Evers and I. Svetlik (eds), *New Welfare Mixes in Care for the Elderly* (vol. 3) (Vienna: European Centre for Social Welfare Policy and Research).

EVERS, A. and I. SVETLIK (eds) (1991) *New Welfare Mixes in Care for the Elderly* (vols 1–3) (Vienna: European Centre for Social Welfare Policy and Research).

EVERS, H. (1981) 'Care or Custody? The Experiences of Women Patients in Long-stay Geriatric Wards', in B. Hutter and G. Williams (eds), *Controlling Women: The Normal and the Deviant* (London: Croom Helm).

FAIRCLOUGH, N. (1989) *Language and Power* (London: Longman).

FEATHERSTONE, M. and M. HEPWORTH (1986) 'New Lifestyles in Old Age?', in C. Phillipson, M. Bernard and P. Strang (eds), *Dependency and Interdependency in Old Age – Theoretical Perspectives and Policy Alternatives* (London: Croom Helm).

FEATHERSTONE, M. and M. HEPWORTH (1990) 'Images of Ageing', in J. Bond and P. Coleman (eds), *Ageing in Society* (London: Sage).

FENNELL, G., C. PHILLIPSON and H. EVERS (1988) *The Sociology of Old Age* (Milton Keynes: Open University Press).

FINCH, J. (1984) 'Community Care: Developing Non-sexist Alternatives', *Critical Social Policy*, 9, pp. 6–18.

FINCH, J. (1989) *Family Obligations* (Cambridge: Polity Press).

FINCH, J. and D. GROVES (1980) 'Community Care and the Family: A Case for Equal Opportunities?', *Journal of Social Policy*, 9 (4), pp. 487–514.

FINCH, J. and D. GROVES (1982) 'By Women for Women: The Care of the Frail Elderly', *Women's Studies International Forum*, 5 (5), pp. 427–38.

FINCH, J. and D. GROVES (eds) (1983) *A Labour of Love* (London: Routledge & Kegan Paul).

FINCH, J. and J. MASON (1990) 'Divorce, Remarriage and Family Obligations', *Sociological Review*, 38 (2), pp. 219–46.

FISCHER, A. (1993) 'Temporary Labour Migration from Central and East Europe: The Case of Germany', in S. Ringen and C. Wallace (eds), *Societies in Transition: East-Central Europe Today* (Prague: Central European University).

FISCHER, D. H. (1978) *Growing Old in America* (New York: Oxford University Press).

FLEETWOOD, J. F. (1980) 'Ireland', in E. Palmore (ed.), *International Handbook on Ageing: Contemporary Developments and Research* (London: Macmillan).

FLOREA, A. (1979) 'Services to the Aged in Italy', in M. I. Teicher, D. Thursz and J. L. Vigilante (eds), *Reaching the Aged: Social Services in Forty-Four Countries* (Beverly Hills, Calif.: Sage).

FLOREA, A. (1980) 'Italy', in E. Palmore (ed.), *International Handbook on Ageing: Contemporary Developments and Research* (London: Macmillan).

FOGARTY, M. P. (1986) *Meeting the Needs of the Elderly* (Dublin: The European Foundation for the Improvement of Living and Working Conditions).

FOSTER, P. (1991) 'Residential Care of Frail Old People: A Possible Reassessment', *Social Policy and Administration*, 25 (2), pp. 108–20.

FOUCAULT, M. (1977) *Discipline and Punish: the Birth of the Prison* (Harmondsworth: Peregrine).

FOULKE, S. R. (1980) *Caring for the Parental Generation* unpublished Master's thesis (Wilmington, Delaware: University of Delaware).

FRIIS, H. (1979) 'The Aged in Denmark', in M. I. Teicher, D. Thursz and J. L. Vigilante (eds), *Reaching the Aged: Social Services in Forty Four Countries* (Beverly Hills, Calif.: Sage).

GARLAND, J. (1990) 'Environment and Behaviour', in J. Bond and P. Coleman (eds), *Ageing in Society* (London: Sage).

GAULLIER, X. (1982) 'The Implications of Greater Activity in Later Life', in M. Fogarty (ed.), *Retirement Policy: The Next Fifty Years* (London: Heinemann).

GEORGE, V. and P. WILDING (1976) *Ideology and Social Welfare* (London: Routledge).

GIDDENS, A. (1991) *Modernity and Self-Identity* (Cambridge: Polity Press).

GILBERT, G. N., A. DALE, S. ARBER, M. EVANDROU and F. LACZKO (1990) 'Resources in Old Age: Ageing and the Life Course' in M. Jeffreys (ed.) *Growing Old in the Twentieth Century* (London: Routledge).

GILLEARD, C. J., A. A. GURKAN and E. GILLEARD (1985) 'Ageing in Turkey: Patterns, Provisions and Prospects' in A. Butler (ed.), *Ageing: Recent Advances and Creative Responses* (London: Croom Helm).

GIORI, D, (1983) 'Old People, Public Expenditure and the System of Social Services: The Italian Case', in A.-M. Guillemard (ed.), *Old Age and the Welfare State* (London: Sage).

GLENDENNING, F. (1993) 'What is Elder Abuse and Neglect?', in P. Decalmer and F. Glendenning (eds), *The Mistreatment of Elderly People* (London: Sage).

GODLOVE, C., L. RICHARD and G. RODWELL (1982) *Time for Change: An Observation Study of Elderly People in Four Different Care Environments* (Sheffield: Joint Unit for Social Services Research).

GOFFMAN, E. (1968) *Asylums* (Harmondsworth: Penguin).

GOFFMAN, E. (1971) *The Presentation of the Self in Everyday Life* (Harmondsworth: Penguin).

GOFFMAN, E. (1975) *Frame Analysis* (Harmondsworth: Peregrine).

GREEN, H. (1988) *General Household Survey 1985: Informal Carers* (London: HMSO).

GROVES, D. (1987) 'Women and Occupational Pension Provision: Past and Future', in S. di Gregorio (ed.), *Social Gerontology: New Directions* (London: Croom Helm).

GROVES, D. and J. FINCH (1985) 'Old Boy, Old Girl', in E. Brook and A. Davis (eds), *Women, the Family and Social Work* (London: Tavistock).

GRUMAN, G. J. (1978) 'Cultural Origins of Present-day "Age-ism": The Modernization of the Life Cycle', in S. F. Spicker, K. M. Woodward and D. D. van Tassel (eds), *Aging and the Elderly: Humanistic Perspectives in Gerontology* (Atlantic Highlands, N. J.: Humanities Press).

GRUNDY, E. (1989) 'Longitudinal Perspectives on the Living Arrangements of the Elderly', in D. Jerrome (ed.), *Growing Old in the Twentieth Century* (London: Routledge & Kegan Paul).

GRUNDY, E. and A. HARROP (1992) 'Demographic Aspects of Ageing in Europe', in L. Davies (ed.), *The Coming of Age in Europe* (London: Age Concern).

GUILLEMARD, A.-M. (1981) 'Old Age, Retirement and the Social Class Structure', in T. K. Hareven (ed.), *Dying and Life Course Transitions* (New York: Guildford Press).

GUILLEMARD, A.-M. (1983) 'The Making of Old Age Policy in France', in A.-M. Guillemard (ed.), *Old Age and the Welfare State* (London: Sage).

GUPTA, H. (1979) 'Can we De-institutionalise an Institution?', *Concord*, 13, pp. 47–57.

GURKAN, A. A. and C. J. GILLEARD (1987) 'Economic Activity of the Elderly in Turkey: An Analysis of Urban and Rural Populations', in S. di Gregorio (ed.), *Social Gerontology: New Directions* (London: Croom Helm).

HAGESTAD, G. O. (1986) 'Challenges and Opportunities of an Ageing Society', in C. Phillipson, M. Bernard and P. Strang (eds), *Dependency and Interdependency in Old Age – Theoretical Perspectives and Policy Alternatives* (London: Croom Helm).

HALLER, M. (1990) 'The Challenge for Comparative Sociology in the Transformation of Europe', *International Sociology*, 5, pp. 183–204.

HARBERT, W. G. and M. DEXTER (1983) *The Home Help Service* (London: Tavistock).

HARTL, J. (1991) 'social policy, Social care and the case of the eldery in Czechoslovakia in A. Evers and I. Svetlik (eds), *New Welfare Mixes in care for the Elderly* (vol. 1) Vienna: European Center for Social Welfare Policy and Research.

HAVIGHURST, R. (1978) 'Ageing in Western Society' in D. Hobman (ed.), *The Social Challenge of Ageing* (London: Croom Helm).

HEDSTRØM, P. and S. RINGEN (1987) 'Age and income in contemporary society', *Journal of Social Policy*, 16 (2), pp. 227–39.

HENDRICKS, J. and C. D. HENDRICKS (1977) *Aging in Mass Society: Myths and Realities* (Cambridge, Mass.: Winthrop).

HENRARD, J.-C. (1991) 'Care for Elderly People in the European Community', *Social Policy and Administration*, 25 (3), pp. 184–92.

HICKS, C. (1988) *Who Cares?* (London: Virago).

HOKENSTAD, M. C. and L. JOHANSSON (1990) 'Caregiving for the Elderly in Sweden', in D. E. Biegel and A. Blum (eds), *Aging and Caregiving: Theory, Research and Policy* (Beverly Hills, Calif.: Sage).

HOLSTEIN, B. E., P. DUE, G. ALMIND, and E. HOLST (1991) 'The home-help service in Denmark', in A. Jamieson (ed.), *Home Care for Older People in Europe: A Comparison of Policies and Practices* (Oxford University Press).

HOMER, A. and C. GILLEARD (1990) 'Abuse of Elderly People and their Carers', *British Medical Journal*, 301, pp. 1359–62.

HOPPEN, K. T. (1989) *Ireland Since 1880: Conflict and Conformity* (London: Longman).

HÖRL, J. (1992) 'Family Care of the Elderly in Austria', in J. I. Kosberg (ed.), *Family Care of the Elderly* (Newbury Park: Sage).

HOWE, D. (1986) *Social Workers and their Practice in Welfare Bureaucracies* (Aldershot: Gower).

HRYNKIEWICZ, J., J. STAREGA-PIASEK and J. SUPINSKA (1991) 'The Elderly and Social Policy in Poland', in A. Evers and I. Svetlik (eds), *New Welfare Mixes in Care for the Elderly* (vol. 1) (Vienna: European Centre for Social Welfare Policy and Research).

HUET, J. A. and A. FONTAINE (1980) 'France' in E. Palmore (ed.), *International Handbook on Ageing: Contemporary Developments and Research* (London: Macmillan).

HUGMAN, R. (1982) 'Images of the Elderly', *Community Care*, 425, pp. 12–13.

HUGMAN, R. (1987) 'The Personal and the Public in Professional Models of Social Work: A Response to O'Connor and Dalgleish', *British Journal of Social Work*, 17 (1), pp. 71–6.

HUGMAN, R. (1991) *Power in Caring Professions* (London: Macmillan).

HUGMAN, R. (1994) 'Consuming Public Services', in N. Abercrombie, R. Keat and N. Whitely (eds), *The Authority of the Consumer* (London: Routledge).

HUNTER, D. (1986) *Care Delivery Systems for the Elderly* (Bath: Age Care Research Europe).

HUSTON, L. (1991) *Shifts in the Welfare Mix: the Case of Care for the Elderly* (Vienna: European Centre for Social Welfare Policy and Research).

HYDLE, I. (1989) 'Violence Against the Elderly in Western Europe', *Journal of Elder Abuse and Neglect*, 1 (3), pp. 75–87.

International Labour Organisation (1986) *Population Active – 1950–2050* (Geneva: International Labour Organisation).

ISAACS, B. and Y. NEVILLE (1976) *The Measurement of Need in Old People*, Scottish Health Service Studies, 34 (Edinburgh: Scottish Home and Health Department).

ISPA (1976) *Informe Sociológico Sobre la Ancianidad en Cataluña* (Barcelona: ISPA).

ITZIN, C. (1986) 'Ageism Awareness Training: A model for Group Work', in C. Phillipson, M. Bernard and P. Strang (eds), *Dependency and Interdependency in Old Age – Theoretical Perspectives and Policy Alternatives* (London: Croom Helm).

JACK, R. (1991) 'Social Services and the Ageing Population 1970–1990', *Social Policy and Administration*, 25 (4), pp. 284–99.

JAMIESON, A. (1990) 'Informal Care in Europe', in A. Jamieson and R. Illsley (eds), *Contrasting European Policies for the Care of Older People* (Aldershot: Avebury).

JAMIESON, A. (1991a) 'Home-care in Europe: Background and Aims', in A. Jamieson (ed.), *Home Care for Older People in Europe: A Comparison of Policies and Practices* (Oxford: (Oxford University Press).

JAMIESON, A. (1991b) 'Home-care Provision and Allocation', in A. Jamieson (ed.), *Home Care for Older People in Europe: A Comparison of Policies and Practices* (Oxford: Oxford University Press).

JAMIESON, A. (1991c) 'Trends in Home-care Policies', in A. Jamieson (ed.), *Home Care for Older People in Europe: a Comparison of Policies and Practices* (Oxford: Oxford University Press).

JAMIESON, A. (1992) 'Community Care for Older People', in G. Room (ed.), *Towards a European Welfare State?* (Bristol: SAUS).

JANI-LE BRIS, H. (1992) *Prise en Charge Familiale des Dependants Ages* (Paris/ Dublin: CLEIRPPA/European Foundation for the Improvement of Living and Working Conditions).

JEFFERYS, M. and P. THANE (1989) 'Introduction: An Ageing Society and Ageing People', in M. Jefferys (ed.), *Growing Old in the Twentieth Century* (London: Routledge).

JENKS, M. and R. NEWMAN (1978) 'Ageing and the Architect', in D. Hobman (ed.), *The Social Challenge of Ageing* (London: Croom Helm).

JERROME, D. (1990) 'Intimate Relationships', in J. Bond and P. Coleman (eds), *Ageing in Society* (London: Sage).

JOHANSSON, L. (1991) 'Informal Care of the Dependent Elderly at Home: Some Swedish Experiences', *Ageing and Society*, 11 (1), pp. 41–58.

JOHNSON, M. (1976) 'That Was Your Life: A Biographical Approach to Later Life', in J. M. A. Munnichs and W. J. A. van den Heuval (eds), *Dependency or Interdependency in Old Age* (The Hague: Martinus Nijhoff).

JOHNSON, P. and J. FALKINGHAN (1992) *Ageing and Economic Welfare* (London: Sage).

JONES, C. (1985) *Patterns of Social Policy: an Introduction to Comparative Analysis* (London: Tavistock).

JOUVENAL, H. de (1988) *Europe's Ageing Population* (Paris/Guildford: Futuribles/Butterworths).

JYLHÄ, M. and J. JOKELA (1990) 'Individual Experiences as Cultural – A Cross-national Study of Loneliness among the Elderly', *Ageing and Society*, 10 (3), pp. 295–315.

KART, G. (1987) 'The End of Conventional Gerontology?', *Sociology of Health and Illness*, 9, pp. 76–88.

KEMPEN, G. I. J. M. and T. P. B. M. SUURMEIJER (1991) 'Factors Influencing Professional Home Care Utilization among the Elderly', *Social Science and Medicine*, 32 (1), pp. 77–81.

KOSBERG, I. J. (1992) 'An International Perspective on Family Care of the Elderly', in I. J. Kosberg (ed.), *Family Care of the Elderly* (Newbury Park: Sage).

KRAAN, R., J. BALDOCK, B. DAVIES, A. EVERS, L. JOHANSSON, M. KNAPEN, M. THORSLUND and C. TUNISSEN (1991) *Care for the Elderly: Significant Innovations in Three European Countries* (Vienna: Campus Verlag).

KUBISA, T. (1990) 'Care Manager: Rhetoric or Reality?', in I. Allen (ed.), *Care Managers and Care Management* (London: Policy Studies Institute).

KUHN, M. (1986) 'Social and Political Goals for an Ageing Society', in C. Phillipson, M. Bernard and P. Strang (eds), *Dependency and Interdependency in Old Age – Theoretical Perspectives and Policy Alternatives* (London: Croom Helm).

KURRLE, S. E., P. M. SADLER and I. D. CAMERON (1991) 'Elder Abuse – An Australian Case Series', *The Medical Journal of Australia*, 155 (3), pp. 150–3.

LACZKO, F. (1990) 'New Poverty and the Old Poor', *Ageing and Society*, 10 (3), pp. 261–77.

LASLETT, P. (1977) *Family Life and Illicit Love in Earlier Generations: Essays in Historical Sociology* (Cambridge University Press).

LASLETT, P. (1989) *A Fresh Map of Life: the Emergence of the Third Age* (London: Weidenfeld & Nicolson).

LAWSON, R. and B. DAVIES with A. Bebbington (1991) 'The Home-Help Service in England and Wales' in A. Jamieson (ed.) *Home Care for Older People in Europe* (Oxford: Oxford University Press).

LEESON, G., L. HAMBURGER, V. PEDERSON and E. TUFTE (1993) *Travel and Culture: Access to Concessions by Older People in Europe*, V/6247/93-EN (Copenhagen/ Luxembourg: DaneAge/Commission of the European Communities).

LEIRA, A. (1990) 'Coping with Care', in C. Ungerson (ed.), *Gender and Caring: Work and Welfare in Britain and Scandinavia* (Hemel Hempstead: Harvester Wheatsheaf).

LEROUX, T. G. and M. PETRUNIK (1990) 'The Construction of Elder Abuse as a Social Problem – A Canadian Perspective', *International Journal of Health Services*, 20 (4), pp. 651–64.

LEWIS, J., CLAK, D. and MOLGAN, D. (1991) *Whom God Hath Joined Together* (London : Routledge).

LISÓN-TOLOSANA, C. (1976) 'The ethics of inheritance', in J. G. Peristiany (ed.), *Mediterranean Family Structures* (Cambridge University Press).

LITTLE, V. (1979) 'For the Elderly: An Overview of Services in Industrially Developed and Developing Countries', in M. I. Teicher, D. Thursz and J. L. Vigilante (eds), *Reaching the Aged: Social Services in Forty Four Countries* (Beverly Hills, Calif.: Sage).

LOBO, A., T. VENTURA and C. MARCO (1990) 'Psychiatric Morbidity among Residents in a Home for the Elderly in Spain', *International Journal of Geriatric Psychiatry*, 5, pp. 83–91.

LOWY, L. (1979) 'Aging: An Overview of Programs and Trends in the Federal Republic of Germany', in M. I. Teicher, D. Thursz and J. L. Vigilante (eds), *Reaching the Aged: Social Services in Forty Four Countries* (Beverly Hills, Calif.: Sage).

MACFARLANE, A. (1986) *Marriage and Love in England: Modes of Reproduction 1300–1840* (Oxford: Basil Blackwell).

MACLEOD, N. and M. SMITH, (1982) 'A Model of Practice in Field Care', in J. Lishman (ed.), *Developing Services for the Elderly* (Aberdeen: University of Aberdeen).

MARIN, Y. (1992) 'Helping Old People Stay at Home', conference paper presented at Marginalisation of Elderly People (Liverpool: Institute of Human Ageing).

MARSHALL, M. and A. SOMMERVILLE (1983) *New Services for Old People* (University of Liverpool Press/Institute of Human Ageing).

MARTIN, J. P. (1984) *Hospitals in Trouble* (Oxford: Basil Blackwell).
MEANS, R. and R. SMITH (1985) *The Development of Welfare Services for Elderly People* (London: Croom Helm).
MIDDLETON, L. (1987) *So Much for So Few: A View of Sheltered Housing* (2nd edn) (Liverpool University Press/Institute of Human Ageing).
MIDRE, G. and B. SYNAK (1989) 'Between Family and State: Ageing in Poland and Norway', *Ageing and Society*, 9 (3), pp. 241–59.
MILLER, E. J. and G. V. GWYNNE (1972) *A Life Apart* (London: Tavistock).
MILLS, C. W. (1956) *White Collar* (New York: Oxford University Press/Galaxy).
MILLS, C. W. (1970) *The Sociological Imagination* (Harmondsworth: Penguin).
MINEV, D., B. DERMENDJIEVA, and N. MILEVA (1990) 'The Bulgaria Country Profile: The Dynamics of Some Inequalities in Health', *Social Science and Medicine* 31 (8), pp. 837–46.
MINOIS, G. (1989) *History of Old Age* (Cambridge: Polity Press).
MISHRA, R. (1984) *The Welfare State in Crisis* (Brighton: Wheatsheaf).
MORRIS, J. (1992) '"Us" and "them"? Feminist Research, Community Care and Disability', *Critical Social Policy*, 33, pp. 22–39.
MYLES, J. (1983) 'Comparative Public Policies for the Elderly: Frameworks and Resources for Analysis', in A.-M. Guillemard (ed.), *Old Age and the Welfare State* (London: Sage).
NAZARETH, J. M. (1976) *Analyse Régionale du Déclin de la Fécondité de la Population Portugaise* (Leuven: Université Catholique de Leuven).
NIES, H., S. TESTER and J. M. NUIJENS (1991) 'Day Care in the UK and The Netherlands: A Comparative Study', *Ageing and Society*, 11 (3), pp. 245–73.
NIRJE, B. (1976) 'The Normalization Principle', in R. Kugel and A. Shearer (eds), *Changing Patterns of Residential Services for the Mentally Handicapped*, revised edn (Washington, D.C.: President's Committee for the Mentally Retarded).
NOIN, D. and A. WARNES (1987) 'Avant-Propos/Foreword' in D. Noin and A. Warnes (eds) *Personnes Agées at Vieillisment* (Lille: Espaces-Populations-Sociétés).
NORMAN, A. (1980) *Rights and Risk* (London: National Corporation for the Care of Old People).
NORMAN, A. (1985) *Triple Jeopardy: Growing Old in a Second Homeland* (London: Centre for Policy on Ageing).
NORMAN, A. (1987) *Aspects of Ageism: a Discussion Paper* (London: Centre for Policy on Ageing).
NORTON, D. (1992) 'Social Provision for Older People in Europe – in Education and Leisure', in L. Davies (ed.), *The Coming of Age in Europe* (London: Age Concern.
OAKLEY, A. (1974) *The Sociology of Housework* (London: Martin Robertson).
O'CONNOR, J. (1973) *The Fiscal Crisis of the State* (New York: St Martin's Press).
OFFE, C. (1984) *Contradictions of the Welfare State* (trans. J. Keane) (London: Hutchinson).
OLIVER, M. (1990) *The Politics of Disability* (London: Macmillan).
OLSEN, N. T. (1991) *Care for the Elderly: Implementation of Ideas in Aalborg* (Aalborg, Denmark: Crone & Koch).
OPCS (Office of Population Censuses and Surveys) (1988) *Disability Survey I and II* (London: HMSO).
OPCS (Office of Population Censuses and Surveys) (1991) *Population Trends* (London: HMSO).

PAILLAT, P. (1989) 'Recent and Predictable Population Trends', in J. Eekelaar and D. Pearl (eds), *An Ageing World* (Oxford: Clarendon Press).

PALME, J. and A.-C. STÅHLBORG (1993) 'A view from Scandinavia: Reforms in Sweden', *Journal of European Social Policy*, 3 (1), pp. 53–6.

PALMORE, E. (ed.) (1980) *International Handbook on Ageing: Contemporary Developments and Research* (London: Macmillan).

PANTELOURIS, E. M. (1987) *Greece: an Introduction* (Moffat: Blueacre Books).

PARKER, G. (1990) *With Due Care and Attention: A Review of Research on Informal Care* (London: Family Policy Studies Centre).

PARKER, S. R. (1982) *Work and Retirement* (London: George Allen & Unwin).

PARRY, N. and J. PARRY (1979) 'Professionalism, Welfare and the State', in M. Rustin, N. Parry and C. Satyamurti (eds), *Social Work, Welfare and the State* (London: Edward Arnold).

PARSONS, T. (1952) *The Social System* (London: Tavistock).

PEACE, S. (1982) 'The Design of Residential Homes: An Historical Perspective', in K. Judge and I. Sinclair (eds), *Residential Care for Elderly People* (London: HMSO).

PEARSON, G. (1975) *The Deviant Imagination* (London: Macmillan).

PENHALE, B. (1993) 'The Abuse of Older People: Considerations for Practice', *British Journal of Social Work*, 23 (2), pp. 95–112.

PETMESIDOU, M. and L. TSOULOUVIS (1991) 'Aspects of the Changing Political Economy of Urban and Regional Development and Planning: Welfare State and Class Segmentation in Postmodern Europe', paper presented at the 8th Urban Change and Conflict Conference, University of Lancaster.

PFLANCZER, S. I. and B. J. BOGNÁR (1989) 'Care of Elderly People in Hungary Today', *The Gerontologist*, 29 (4), pp. 546–50.

PHILLIPS, M. (1982) 'Separatism or Black control?' in A. Ohri, B. Manning and P. Curno (eds), *Community Work and Racism* (London: Routledge & Kegan Paul).

PHILLIPSON, C. (1982) *Capitalism and the Construction of Old Age* (London: Macmillan).

PHILLIPSON, C. (1990) 'The Sociology of Retirement', in J. Bond and P. Coleman (eds), *Ageing in Society* (London: Sage).

PHILLIPSON, C. (1992) 'Great Britain', in J. I. Kosberg (ed.), *Family Care of the Elderly* (Newbury Park: Sage).

PHILLIPSON, C. and P. STRANG (1985) 'Sheltered Housing: The Warden's View', in A. Butler (ed.), *Ageing: Recent Advances and Creative Responses* (London: Croom Helm).

PHILLIPSON, C. and A. WALKER (1987) 'The Case for a Critical Gerontology', in S. di Gregorio (ed.), *Social Gerontology: New Directions* (London: Croom Helm).

PHILLIPSON, C. and S. BIGGS (1992) *Understanding Elder Abuse* (London: Longman).

PIJL, M. (1991) 'Netherlands', in A. Evers and I. Svetlik (eds), *New Welfare Mixes in Care for the Elderly* (vol. 2) (Vienna: European Centre for Social Welfare Policy and Research).

PIJL, M. (1992) 'Netherlands Policies for Elderly People', *Social Policy and Administration*, 26 (3), pp. 201–8.

PITAUD, P. and R. VERCAUTEREN with B. DHERBY (1991) 'France', in Evers, A. and Svetlik, I. (eds), *New Welfare Mixes in Care for the Elderly* (vol. 3) (Vienna: European Centre for Social Welfare Policy and Research).

PITKEATHLEY, J. (1989) *It's My Duty Isn't It?* (London: Souvenir Press).
PITSIOU, E. (1986) *Life Styles of Older Athenians*, Vol. 1 (Athens: National Centre of Social Research).
POWER, B. (1980) *Old and Alone in Ireland* (Dublin: Society of St Vincent de Paul).
PRITCHARD, J. (1992) *The Abuse of Elderly People* (London: Jessice Kingsley).
PSYCHOGIOS, D. (1987) *Dowries, Taxes, Raisins and Bread: Economy and Family in Rural Greece in the Nineteenth Century* (in Greek) (Athens: National Centre of Social Research).
QUADAGNO, J. (1982) *Aging in Early Industrial Society: Work, Family and Social Policy in Nineteenth Century England* (New York: Academic Press).
QURESHI, H. and WALKER, A. (1989) *The Caring Relationship* (London: Macmillan).
RAMON, S. (1991) 'Policy Issues', in S. Ramon (ed.), *Beyond Community Care* (London: Macmillan).
RASMUSSEN, B. L. (1991) *The Danish Elderly Care System* (Aalborg, Denmark: Crone & Koch).
REIN, M. (1976) *Social Science and Public Policy* (Harmondsworth: Penguin).
RHEIN, C. (1987) 'Transformations des structures urbaines et vieillissement démographique dans l'agglomération Parisienne, 1954–1982', in D. Nion and A. Warnes (eds), *Personnes Agées et Vieillissment* (Lille: Espaces-Populations-Sociétés).
ROBINSON, F. and N. GREGSON (1992) 'The "Underclass": A Class Apart?', *Critical Social Policy*, 34, pp. 38–51.
ROBOLIS, S. (1993) 'A View from the South: Reforms in Greece', *Journal of European Social Policy*, 3 (1), pp. 56–9.
ROONEY, B. (1987) *Racism and Resistance to Change* (Liverpool: Merseyside Area Profile Group).
ROSE, R. (1993) 'Who Needs Social Protection in East Europe? A Constrained Empirical Analysis of Romania', in S. Ringen and C. Wallace (eds), *Societies in Transition: East-Central Europe Today* (Prague: Central European University).
ROSE, R. and R. SHIRATORI (eds) (1986) *The Welfare State East and West* (Oxford University Press).
ROSENMAYR, L. (1969) 'Soziologie des Älters', in R. König (ed.), *Handbuch der Empirischen Soziologie* (vol. 2) (Stuttgart: Enke).
ROSENMAYR, L. (1972) 'The Elderly in Austrian Society', in D. O. Cowgill and L. D. Holmes (eds), *Aging and Modernization* (New York: Appleton–Century–Crofts).
ROSENMAYR, L. and E. KÖCEIS (1963) 'Propositions for a Sociological Theory of Ageing and the Family', *International Social Science Journal*, XV (3), pp. 410–26.
ROWBOTHAM, S. (1974) *Hidden From History: 300 Years of Women's Oppression and the Fight Against It* (London: Pluto Press).
RUSICA, M., I. HOJNIC-ZUPANC and I. SVETLIK (1991) 'Yugoslavia', in A. Evers and I. Svetlik (eds), *New Welfare Mixes in Care for the Elderly* (vol. 1) (Vienna: European Centre for Social Welfare Policy and Research).
SAIFULLAH KHAN, V. (1977) 'The Pakistanis: Mipur Villagers at Home and in Bradford', in J. L. Watson (ed.), *Between Two Cultures* (Oxford: Basil Blackwell).

SAINSBURY, E., S. NIXON and D. PHILLIPS (1982) *Social Work in Focus* (London: Routledge & Kegan Paul).

SALTMAN, R. B. (1991) 'Emerging trends in the Swedish health system', *International Journal of Health Services*, 21 (4), pp. 615–23.

SANIDAD Y SEGURIDAD (1981) *Introducción a la Gerontología Social* (Madrid: Servicio de Publicaciones del Ministerio de Trabajo).

SANT CASSIA, P., with C. BADA (1992) *The Making of the Modern Greek Family* (Cambridge University Press).

SCOTT SMITH, D. (1982) 'Historical Change in the Household Structure of the Elderly in Economically Developed Societies', in P. N. Stearns (ed.), *Old Age in Pre-Industrial Society* (New York: Holmes & Meier).

SCULL, A. (1979) *Museums of Madness* (London: Allen Lane).

SCULL, A. (1984) *Decarceration* (2nd edn) (Cambridge: Polity Press).

SEALE, C. (1990) 'Caring for People Who Die: The Experience of Family and Friends', *Ageing and Society*, 10 (4), pp. 413–28.

SERVIAN, R., T. REGNART and M. JAGER (eds), (1990) *Room to Care* (Birmingham: BASW).

SHANAS, E., P. TOWNSEND, D. WEDDERBURN, H. FRIIS, P. MILHOJ and J. STEHOUWER (1968) *Old People in Three Industrial Societies* (London: Routledge & Kegan Paul).

SHEPPARD, H. L. and L. C. MULLINS, (1989) 'A Comparative Examination of Perceived Income Inadequacy among Young and Old in Sweden and the United States', *Ageing and Society*, 9 (3), pp. 223–39.

SIIM, B. (1990) 'Women and the Welfare State: Between Private and Public Dependence', in C. Ungerson (ed.), *Gender and Caring: Work and Welfare in Britain and Scandinavia* (Hemel Hempstead: Harvester Wheatsheaf).

SILVERMAN, P. and R. J. MAXWELL (1982) 'Cross-cultural Variation in the Status of Old People', in P. N. Stearns (ed.), *Old Age in Pre-Industrial Society* (New York: Holmes & Meier).

SIMMONS, L. (1945) *The Role of the Aged in Primitive Society* (New Haven, Conn.: Yale University Press).

SMITH, S. R. (1982) 'Growing Old in an Age of Transition', in P. N. Stearns (ed.), *Old Age in Pre-Industrial Society* (New York: Holmes & Meier).

SMOLIC-KRKOVIC, D. N. (1979) 'Aging in Yugoslavia', in M. I. Teicher, D. Thursz and J. L. Vigilante (eds), *Reaching the Aged: Social Services in Forty Four Countries* (Beverly Hills, Calif.: Sage).

Social Europe (1991) 'Immigration to Southern EC Members', 1/91 (Brusells: Commission of the European Community).

Social Services Inspectorate (1992) *Confronting Elder Abuse* (London: HMSO).

SONTAG, S. (1978) 'The Double Standard of Ageing', in V. Carver and P. Liddiard (eds), *An Ageing Population: A Reader and Sourcebook* (Sevenoaks: Hodder and Stoughton/Open University Press).

STANG, G. (1986) *Elder Abuse Documented in Norway* (Oslo: Rikhospitalet, Institutt for Sosialmedisin).

STATHOPOULOS, P. and A. AMERA (1992) 'Care of the Elderly in Greece', in I. J. Kosberg (ed.), *Family Care of the Elderly* (Newbury Park: Sage).

STEARNS, P. N. (1977) *Old Age in European Society: The Case of France* (London: Croom Helm).

STEENVOORDEN, M. A., F. G. VAN DER PLAS and N. G. DE BOER (1992) *Family Care of the Older Elderly: Casebook of Initiatives* (Utrecht/Dublin: Nederlands Instituut voor Zorg en Welzijn/European Foundation for the Improvement of Living and Working Conditions).

STEINMETZ, S. K. (1988) *Duty Bound: Elder Abuse and Family Care* (Beverly Hills, Calif.: Sage).

SVETLIK, I. (1991) 'The future of Welfare Pluralism in the Post-Communist Countries', in A. Evers and I. Svetlik (eds), *New Welfare Mixes in Care for the Elderly*, (vol.1) (Vienna: European Centre for Social Welfare Policy and Research).

SUNDSTRØM, G. (1986) 'Family and State: Trends in the Care of the Aged in Sweden', *Ageing and Society*, 6 (2), pp. 169–96.

SYNAK, B. (1987a) 'The Elderly in Poland: An Overview of Selected Problems and Changes', in S. di Gregorio (ed.), *Social Gerontology: New Directions* (London: Croom Helm).

SYNAK, B. (1987b) 'The Elderly in Poland' *Ageing and Society*, 7 (1), pp. 19–35.

SZÉMAN, Z. (1992) 'New Policy for the Old', in B. Deacon (ed.), *Social Policy, Social Justice and Citizenship in Eastern Europe* (Aldershot: Avebury).

SZÉMAN, Z. and E. SIK (1991) 'Why Social Innovations are Needed in Care for the Elderly: The Case of Hungary', in A. Evers and I. Svetlik (eds), *New Welfare Mixes in Care for the Elderly* (vol. 1) (Vienna: European Centre for Social Welfare Policy and Research).

SZÉMAN, Z. and V. GÁTHY (1993) 'The Voluntary Sector in the Welfare Mix', *Journal of European Social Policy*, 3 (2), pp. 119–129.

TAWNEY, R. H. (1926) *Religion and the Rise of Capitalism* (London: Murray).

TAYLOR, D. (1989) 'Citizenship and Social Power', *Critical Social Policy*, 26, pp. 19–31.

TEICHER, M. I., D. THURSZ and J. L. VIGILANTE (eds) (1979) *Reaching the Aged: Social Services in Forty Four Countries* (Beverly Hills, Calif.: Sage).

TEPEROGLOU, A. (1980) 'Open Care for the Elderly – Greece', in A. Amann (ed.), *Open Care for the Elderly in Seven European Countries* (Oxford: Pergamon Press).

TEPEROGLOU, A., with E. KINIA, M. PAPAKOSTA and M. TZORTZOPOULOU (1990) *Evaluation of the Contribution of Open Care Centres for the Elderly* (in Greek) (Athens: National Centre of Social Research).

TENTORI, T. (1976) 'Social Class and Family in a South Italy Town: Matera', in J. G. Peristiany (ed.), *Mediterranean Family Structures* (Cambridge: Cambridge University Press).

TESTER, S. and B. MEREDITH (1987) *Ill Informed?* (London: Policy Studies Institute).

THANE, P. (1982) *The Foundations of the Welfare State* (London: Longman).

THANE, P. (1983) 'The History of Provision for the Elderly to 1929', in D. Jerrome (ed.), *Ageing in Modern Society* (New York: St Martin's Press).

THORSLUND, M. (1991) 'The Increasing Number of Very Old People Will Change the Swedish Model of the Welfare State', *Social Science and Medicine*, 32 (4), pp. 455–64.

THORSLUND, M. and L. JOHANSSON (1987) 'Elderly People in Sweden: Current Realities and Future Plans', *Ageing and Society*, 7 (3), pp. 345–55.

TINKER, A. (1981) *The Elderly in Modern Society* (London: Longman).

TITMUSS, R. (1963) *Essays on the Welfare State* (2nd edn) (London: George Allen & Unwin).

TORKINGTON, N. P. K. (1983) *The Racial Politics of Health* (Liverpool: Merseyside Area Profile Group).

TORNSTAM, L. (1989) 'Abuse of the Elderly in Denmark and Sweden. Result from a Population Study', *Journal of Elder Abuse and Neglect*, 1 (1), pp. 35–44.

TOURAINE, A. (1969) *La Société Post-industrielle* (Paris: Denoël).

TOWNSEND, P. (1958) 'A Society for People', in N. McKenzie (ed.), *Conviction* (London: MacGibbon & Kee).

TOWNSEND, P. (1979) *Poverty in the United Kingdom* (Harmondsworth: Penguin).

TOWNSEND, P. and D. WEDDERBURN (1965) *The Aged and the Welfare State* (London: G. Bell and Sons).

TOWNSEND, P. and N. DAVIDSON (1982) *Inequalities in Health* (Harmondsworth: Penguin).

TRIANTAFILLOU, J. H., A. AMERA and A. GEORGIADOU (1986) *Health and Use of Services by the Elderly in Rural Greece 1985–6* (unpublished report) (Athens: Center of Studies of Age-Related Changes in Man).

TRIANTAFILLOU, J. H. and E. MESTHENEOS (1990) *Pathways to Care: A Study of Greek Elderly People and Their Use of Hospital Emergency Department Services* (unpublished report) (Athens: Center of Studies of Age-Related Changes in Man).

UNGERSON, C. (1983) 'Why Do Women Care?', in J. Finch and D. Groves (eds), *A Labour of Love: Women, Work and Caring* (London: Routledge & Kegan Paul).

UNGERSON, C. (1987) *Policy is Personal* (London: Tavistock).

UNGERSON, C. (1990) 'The language of care', in C. Ungerson (ed.), *Gender and Caring: Work and Welfare in Britain and Scandinavia* (Hemel Hempstead: Harvester Wheatsheaf).

United Nations (1986) *World Population Prospects* (New York: United Nations).

United Nations (1992) *Demographic Yearbook 1990* (New York: United Nations).

URRY, J. (1990) *The Tourist Gaze* (London: Sage).

VICTOR, C. R. (1985) 'Welfare Benefits and the Elderly', in A. Butler (ed.), *Ageing: Recent Advances and Creative Responses* (London: Croom Helm).

VICTOR, C. R. (1987) *Old Age in Modern Society* (London: Chapman Hall).

Vierter Familienbericht (1986) *Der Situation der Älteren Menschen in der Familie* (Bonn: Der Bundesminister für Jugend, Familie, Frauen und Gesundheit).

WÆRNESS, K. (1990) 'Informal and Formal Care in Old Age', in C. Ungerson (ed.), *Gender and Caring: Work and Welfare in Britain and Scandinavia* (Hemel Hempstead: Harvester Wheatsheaf).

WAGNE, G. (1990) *A Positive Choice*, vol. 1 (London: HMSO).

WALKER, A. (1981) 'Towards a Political Economy of Old age', *Ageing and Society*, 1 (1), 73–94.

WALKER, A. (1986a) 'Pensions and the Production of Poverty in Old Age', in C. Phillipson and A. Walker (eds), *Ageing and Social Policy* (Aldershot: Gower).

WALKER, A. (1986b) 'The Politics of Ageing in Britain', in C. Phillipson, M. Bernard and P. Strang (eds), *Dependency and Interdependency in Old Age – Theoretical Perspectives and Policy Alternatives* (London: Croom Helm).

WALKER, A. (1987) 'The Poor Relation: Poverty Among Old Women', in C. Glendinning and J. Millar (eds), *Women and Poverty in Britain* (Brighton: Wheatsheaf).

WALKER, A. (1990) 'Poverty and Inequality in Old Age', in J. Bond and P. Coleman (eds), *Ageing in Society* (London: Sage).

WALTON, R. (1982) *Social Work 2000* (London: Longman).

WARNES, A. (1987a) 'Population, Geography and Ageing in Britain and France: Research and Applied Issues', in D. Noin and A. Warnes (eds), *Personnes Agées et Vieillissment* (Lille: Espaces-Populations-Sociétés).

WARNES, A. (1987b) 'The Distribution of the Elderly Population of Great Britain', in D. Nion and A. Warnes (eds), *Personnes Agées et Vieillissment* (Lille: Espaces-Populations-Sociétés).

WEBER, M. (1930) (trans. T. Parsons) *The Protestant Ethic and the Spirit of Capitalism* (London: George Allen & Unwin).

WELCH, R. D. and S. H. BOYD (1990) *Report of an Inspection of Adult Placement Schemes in Solihull* (Birmingham: Social Services Inspectorate).

WENGER, G. C. (1984) *The Supportive Relationship: Coping with Old Age* (London: George Allen & Unwin).

WENGER, G. C. (1988) *Old People's Health and Experiences of the Caring Services* (Liverpool University Press/Insitute of Human Ageing).

WENGER. G. C. (1989) *Elderly Carers: the Need for Appropriate Intervention* (Bangor: Centre for Social Policy Research and Development).

WILLCOCKS, D. (1982) 'Residential Homes as Community Care: A Future Place for Old People's Homes in the Community They Serve', in K. Judge and I. Sinclair (eds), *Residential Care for Elderly People* (London: HMSO).

WILLCOCKS, D. (1983) 'Stereotypes of Old Age: The Case of Yugoslavia', in D. Jerrome (ed.), *Ageing in Modern Society* (London: Croom Helm).

WILLCOCKS, D., S. PEACE and L. KELLAHER (1987) *Private Lives in Public Places* (London: Tavistock).

WILLIAMS, J. (1990) 'Elders from Black and Minority Ethnic Communities', in I. Sinclair, R. Parker, D. Leat and J. Williams (eds), *The Kaleidoscope of Care* (London: HMSO/National Institute of Social Work).

WILLIAMSON, J. B. and F. C. PAMPEL (1991) 'Ethnic Politics, Colonial Legacy and Old Age Security Policy', *Journal of Ageing Studies*, 5 (1), pp. 19–44.

WILLMOTT, P. and M. YOUNG (1962) *Family and Kinship in East London* (Harmondsworth: Penguin).

WILSON, B. (1976) *The Contemporary Transformations of Religion* (Oxford: Oxford University Press).

WING, J. and G. BROWN (1970) *Institutionalism and Schizophrenia* (Cambridge: Cambridge University Press).

WISENSALE, S. K. (1988) 'Generational Equity and Intergenerational Politics', *The Gerontologist*, 28 (6), pp. 773–8.

WOLF, R. S. and K. A. PILLEMER (1989) *Helping Elderly Victims: The Reality of Elder Abuse* (New York: Columbia University Press).

ZAPF, W. (1986) 'Developments, Structure and Prospects of the German Social State', in R. Rose and R. Shiratori (eds), *The Welfare State East and West* (Oxford: Oxford University Press).

ZARRAS, J. (1980) 'Greece', in E. Palmore (ed.), *International Handbook on Ageing: Contemporary Developments and Research* (London: Macmillan).

Index

194 *Index*